THE One-Minute Workout

THE One-Minute Workout

REAL DEAL FITNESS AND NUTRITION

Andrew Oye, CPT & Robert Dothard, CPT

Want Real Results?
Got a Minute?
Get Real!

Hilton Publishing
1630 45th Street, Suite 103
Munster, IN 46321
219-922-4868
www.hiltonpub.com

Copyright © 2008 by Andrew Oye and Robert Dothard. All rights reserved.

No portion of this book may be reproduced, stored in a retrieval system or transmitted in any form or by any means—electronic, mechanical, photocopy, recording, or any other—except for brief quotation in printed reviews, without prior permission of the authors/publishers.

Printed in the United States of America

10 9 8 7 6 5 4 3 2 1

Photography Credits and Respective Copyrights:
Authors' photos and all resistance training exercise demonstration photography by Shawn Dowdell.
All stretching exercise demonstration photography by Jamo Nezzar.
Pages: front cover, i, 4, 5, 10, 11, 15, 18, 21, 22, back cover
Stock photography courtesy of www.morguefile.com
Pages: title page, ii, 1-3, 6-9, 25, 26, 33, 34, 37, 40 (top left, top right), 41, 48, 49, 53, 56-60, closing page
Stock photography courtesy of www.freeimages.co.uk
Pages: 40 (bottom left, bottom right), 52

Creative Art Direction:
Interior Content Creative Direction, Layout and Design by Andrew Oye
Exterior Cover Creative Direction, Layout and Design by Andrew Oye

Library of Congress Cataloging-in-Publication Data

Dothard, Robert.
   The one-minute workout : real deal fitness & nutrition / by Robert Dothard, Andrew Oye.
     p. cm.
   ISBN 978-0-9800649-2-6
    1. Physical fitness. 2. Exercise. 3. Nutrition. 4. Health. I. Oye, Andrew. II. Title.
   RA781.D59 2008
   613.7—dc22
                                    2008017468

DISCLAIMER: The information contained in this book is for educational purposes only. No approval, agreement, support or warranty is given or implied concerning the information; therefore, the reader/end user exercises his or her own risk by utilizing this information. As individuals and results are unique, the authors make no representations, warranties or guarantees of any kind about the results you may achieve from following the exercise, nutrition or supplementation programs or recommendations. The information contained herein is not medical advice and is not intended to replace the advice or attention of healthcare professionals. Consult your physician or healthcare provider before beginning or making any changes to your exercise, nutrition or supplementation program. Consult your physician or healthcare provider, particularly if you use prescription or over-the-counter medicines; if you are being treated by a professional for any chronic or medical condition; or if you seek diagnosis and treatment of illness and injuries, or for advice regarding medications. The U.S. Food and Drug Administration has not evaluated the statements in this book pertaining to the effects of nutrition or nutritional supplements. None of these supplements are intended to diagnose, treat, cure or prevent any condition or disease. The information contained in this book is an expression of the authors' opinions and should not be interpreted as definitive scientific conclusions of any kind. Therefore, the authors are not liable for any damages (compensatory, direct, indirect, consequential, physical, medical or otherwise) arising out of or in connection with the use of this information by any reader/end user.

DEDICATION

THE ONE-MINUTE WORKOUT: Real Deal Fitness & Nutrition is dedicated to all of you who have struggled with fitness, to all of you who are now determined to achieve new fitness goals, and to those of you who will eventually spread the REAL DEAL gospel to those who don't yet know what you now know.

ACKNOWLEDGMENTS

Immense thanks to our various clients, because the fitness challenges and triumphs that you shared with us while working together inspired this book. Thanks to our fitness models who appear in the exercise demonstration photographs in *The REAL DEAL Training Guide*: Erik Berger, Natasha Richardson, Sarah Krippner, Mona Liza Reyes and Helen Grace Olivares. Thanks to photographer Shawn Dowdell (www.shawndowdell.com) and to makeup artist Synthe Fleming (www.syntheonline.com) for lending your creative talents to the photography sessions. Thanks to Roman Fortin of The Forum Athletic Club for use of your wonderful facility (www.theforumathleticclub.com). Special thanks to our collective family, friends and supporters who cheered us on along our journey to the completion of this project.

CONTENTS

Introduction • ONE MINUTE = ONE LIFETIME xi

Chapter 1 • The REAL DEAL Four-Step Formula 1

REAL DEAL FITNESS • THE TRAINING GUIDE

Welcome to REAL DEAL Training

Chapter 2 • The REAL DEAL Workout Drills 5

Chapter 3 • The ONE-MINUTE Workout Program 9

REAL DEAL NUTRITION • THE EATING GUIDE

Welcome to REAL DEAL Eating

Chapter 4 • The REAL DEAL Dietary Guidelines 23

Chapter 5 • The REAL DEAL Meal Plan 33

Chapter 6 • REAL DEAL Wellness 37

Conclusion—One Lifetime = One Journey 43

REAL DEAL TRAINING GUIDE RESOURCES

Stretching Exercises: Demonstrations & Descriptions 47

Resistance Training Exercises: Demonstrations & Descriptions 53

Cardiovascular/Aerobic Exercises: Descriptions 88

REAL DEAL Training Log 90

REAL DEAL Personal Progress Log 91

REAL DEAL EATING GUIDE RESOURCES

More or Less List 95

How to Read Nutrition Facts Labels 96

The Glycemic Index 98

The Difference Between LDL and HDL Cholesterol 99

5 REAL Keys to Weight Management 100

The Real Smart Shopper's Grocery Checklist 101

REAL DEAL Eating Log 102

About the Authors 103

INTRODUCTION

ONE MINUTE = ONE LIFETIME

Starting a fitness program is a hurdle many people face. **THE ONE-MINUTE WORKOUT: Real Deal Fitness and Nutrition** is a results-oriented health and fitness guide to help you jump that hurdle. With basic yet effective training and eating programs that can be used to change your body and health habits, this is your guidebook on the road to the "best you."

Your guides on this journey are Fitness Coaches Andrew Oye, CPT, and Robert Dothard, CPT. Our duty is to coach you toward improving your fitness and sticking with a healthy lifestyle program.

Our philosophy is built upon the R.E.A.L. Concept, monitoring four basic elements of health:

1. Rest (Repair, Recuperation, Relaxation, Stress Relief, "You Time")
2. Exercise (Aerobic and Resistance Training, Cardiovascular and Muscular Health)
3. Appetite (Diet, Nutrition, Supplementation, Moderation)
4. Lifestyle (Balance, Longevity, Spirituality, Habits, Quality of Life)

We define wellness as a balance of rest, exercise, appetite and lifestyle for the best quality of life. This guidebook opens with *The REAL DEAL Four-Step Formula,* an equation of four steps that breakdown the path to wellness:

Wake up!
Get real!
Take action!
Get results!

When it comes to taking action, *The REAL DEAL Training Guide* lays out the resistance training, cardiovascular activity and stretching exercises you can do to act on the fitness goals you've set for yourself. The guide fully explains the stages you'll encounter in setting and reaching those goals called *The REAL DEAL Workout Drills,* or *"The 6 W's"*

Want it!
Warm up!
Workout!
Work through it!

Wind down!
Work your way up!

Then we delve into *The One-Minute Workout* program, a simple plan based on a one-minute principle: train each major muscle group with one minute of resistance exercise using moderate resistance split by one-minute aerobic intervals.

To supplement and complement your training, refer to The REAL DEAL Eating Guide for sensible nutritional advice. The foundation of the Eating Guide is based on 7 rules referred to as The REAL DEAL Dietary Guidelines:

For your total health plan, refer to the positive lifestyle habits in our discussion on REAL DEAL Wellness in the final chapter.

Rule 1: Mix It Up!
Rule 2: Get Carb Smart!
Rule 3: Avoid Bad Fat!
Rule 4: Burn Your Food!
Rule 5: Limit Your Booze!
Rule 6: Skip The Sugar!
Rule 7: Shake The Salt!

The Living Guide focuses on the areas of life.

Throughout the book, be on the lookout for REAL DEAL Training, Nutrition and Wellness Principles. These are convenient tips to which you can continually refer to help you with your lifestyle renovation process.

Your mission is to get fit and to stay fit. Results start when you do, so get started now! No need to worry. With **THE ONE-MINUTE WORKOUT**, it will only take a minute.

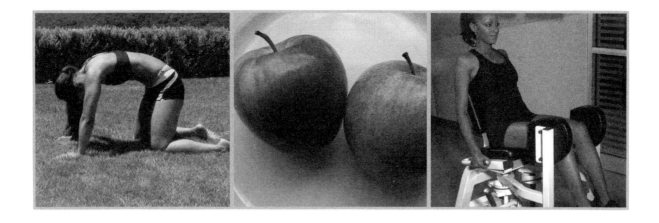

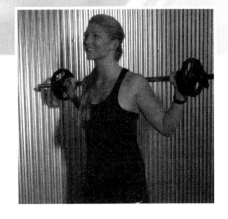

CHAPTER 1
THE REAL DEAL FOUR-STEP FORMULA

There are four steps you can apply to your life immediately to understand the necessity of exercise and good nutrition. Collectively, these steps are called *The REAL DEAL Four-Step Formula*:

WAKE UP + GET REAL + TAKE ACTION = GET RESULTS

WAKE UP!

Waking up means "facing facts."

Fact: More than a third of America is overweight or obese. According the Centers for Disease Control and Prevention, in the past 30 years, the overweight and obese population has increased sharply among both adults and children. Between 1976–1980 and 2003–2004, obesity among adults aged 20–74 years increased from 15.0% to 32.9%. The number of overweight young people increased from 5.0% to 13.9% for those aged 2–5 years, 6.5% to 18.8% for those aged 6–11 years, and 5.0% to 17.4% for those aged 12–19 years. Because people who are obese are at increased risk for heart disease, high blood pressure, diabetes, arthritis-related disabilities, and some cancers the estimated total cost of obesity in the United States in 2000 was about $117 billion (cdc.gov).

These staggering statistics become real in the faces of the many obese and/or unhealthy people in our workplaces, in our families, and in our very own mirrors. It's time for a wake-up call!

Wake-up calls usually come to us in one of three forms:

1. Medical diagnosis: an assessment of your physical condition made by a medical professional
2. Lifestyle diagnosis: an assessment of your physical appearance and conditioning based on your mirror, ill-fitting clothes, limitations on former or current physical activities, etc.
3. Confessional diagnosis: an assessment of your physical appearance based on an honest personal opinion or the opinions of others

Whether it's a high blood pressure diagnosis, ill-fitting old blue jeans, or your spouse's admission that you don't strut quite like you used to, once you receive the call, wake up and respond!

GET REAL!

Getting real means "assessing then addressing."

Assess your health status, using tools that determine body weight (scale, caliper, medical physical). and then commit to making the necessary changes to address areas of concern. Fitness gadget hype ads, diet gimmicks, and instant weight-loss infomercials can be overwhelming. Often, commercial media and marketing feeds us an unhealthy diet of misinformation. False promises of instant, easy or permanent results can leave dashed hopes of better bodies hanging off our waistlines.

Advertising tells us we're incomplete and offers us "quick fixes" for our problems. If they offered the cure, they'd be out of business. If you're not satisfied with the reflection in the mirror, ask yourself: "Have I done what's required for a fit and healthy body?" If not, what needs to be done about the health habits that have made your body what it is today?

TAKE ACTION!

Taking action means "doing not saying."

You used to do as the coach said, remember? Everyone has been required to enroll in Physical Education (PE) classes at one point in his or her life; unfortunately, many tend to forget those grade-school lessons when they no longer have coaches encouraging (or, in some cases, forcing) them to exercise.

Well, PE class is back in session. Stop saying what you want to do. Start doing what you need to do. To help you to take steps toward a more action-driven lifestyle, refer to *The REAL DEAL Training Guide* (page 3). The One-Minute Workout is a program in which almost everyone can participate and succeed. Simply identify your fitness level, select the relevant workout programs and get to work. Taking real, deliberate action to improve the way you look and feel yields positive changes, because action determines the difference between where you are and where you want to be.

GET RESULTS!

Getting results means "earning happiness."

We all deserve to by happy, right? Actually, we're only guaranteed the right to the "pursuit of happiness." Pursuing nutrition and exercise with diligence is how you earn the satisfaction you may feel you deserve.

The threat of obesity, the lure of weight-loss misinformation and the excuse of "limited time" are the evils that thwart our goals. Boldly take on these opponents with the advice in this manual and claim your prize—the desired results of an improved physique, a healthier eating plan, and a more active lifestyle.

Remember these three essential truths:

> The results you get are in direct correlation to the action you take.
> Results start when you do.
> Results stop when you do.

An additional reward of hard work is the knowledge that you earn any success you attain. Together, we can win the race of life. The championship trophies will be millions of fit, healthy bodies—one for each of us.

REAL DEAL FITNESS
THE TRAINING GUIDE

WELCOME TO REAL DEAL TRAINING

Now that we have reviewed *The REAL DEAL Four-Step Formula* for launching your fitness journey, let's explore a major component in your tool kit: training and exercise. Welcome to REAL DEAL Training.

Effective training means practicing consistent exercise habits for proper weight management and good health. *The REAL DEAL Training Guide* contains exercise programs, tips and advice that can help change your body in a real way.

We open the guide with *The REAL DEAL Workout Drills*. These drills are the six key stages you will follow to add and keep exercise in your daily life. Exercise includes stretching, resistance training, and cardiovascular/aerobic activity.

What is stretching? Stretching is deliberately elongating specific muscles or muscle groups to their fullest length to improve the elasticity, reaffirm muscle tone and reduce soreness.

What is resistance training? Resistance training is the extension and contraction of muscles working against opposing force (resistance). The resistance can be weights (on a barbell, dumbbell or machine), elastic bands/tubing, or your own body weight.

What is cardiovascular/aerobic activity? Aerobic exercise in an activity (like jogging or jumping rope) that improves the body's oxygen consumption and strengthens the muscles involved in respiration, namely the heart and lungs.

Your new or existing exercise routine can be also be enhanced by the tips included in this guide. These include:

Basic Stretching Exercise Tips
Basic Resistance Training Tips
Basic Cardiovascular/Aerobic Training Tips

Lastly, we close with *REAL DEAL Training Principles*. These principles are a shorthand way to summarize everything in the training guide and a convenient way to remember our recommendations. Ready? Set? Let's train.

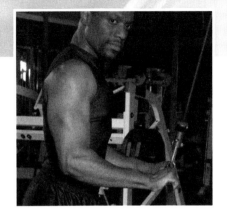

CHAPTER 2

THE REAL DEAL WORKOUT DRILLS

THE REAL DEAL WORKOUT DRILLS • "THE 6 W'S"

Whether you are a Novice, Intermediate or Advanced exerciser, your approach to your workout program should include six steps that we call *The REAL DEAL Workout Drills* or *"The 6 W's"*:

Drill 1: Want It!
Drill 2: Warm Up!
Drill 3: Work Out!
Drill 4: Work Through It!
Drill 5: Wind Down!
Drill 6: Work Your Way Up!

Let's explore these drills for those of you at all fitness levels: the Novice exerciser, who needs to jumpstart a fitness program; the Intermediate exerciser, who wants to elevate an existing fitness program; and the Advanced exerciser, who wants to revamp or remix an ongoing fitness program. Pick your level and proceed.

DRILL 1 • Want It!

NOVICE: When starting a fitness regime, setting goals is key. The way to jumpstart your program is to take a minute to consider what you want from your body and how exercise can help you achieve the goals you have for your body. When you walk into the gym or wherever else you choose to exercise, know what you want to achieve each day and in the long run. Use *The REAL DEAL Training Log* included in this guidebook (page 90) to keep track of your objectives and achievements.

INTERMEDIATE and ADVANCED: After you have committed to exercising regularly, goal setting remains important to maintaining results and pursuing new goals. At your sessions, know what you want to achieve each day, while keeping in mind your long-term goals. Use *The REAL DEAL Training Log* (page 90) to keep track of your objectives and achievements.

DRILL 2 • Warm Up!

NOVICE, INTERMEDIATE and ADVANCED: No matter your fitness level, before you begin exercising, warm up with comfortable stretches and/or light aerobic activity to prepare your muscles for more vigorous activity. Use stretches to awaken your muscles, retain muscle elasticity and increase your flexibility.

As you warm up, keep in mind these *Basic Stretching Exercise Tips:*

1. Hold stretches for 10 to 20 seconds or until the tension in a muscle relaxes.
2. Use proper form/technique.
3. Keep spine pressed into the floor when in a lying position.
4. Do not jerk/bounce or force your body beyond what it is capable of.

Refer to the list of *Stretching Exercises* (page 47) complete with demonstrations and descriptions. Perform lower body stretches before training your lower body. Perform upper body stretches before training your upper body.

DRILL 3 • Work Out!

NOVICE, INTERMEDIATE and ADVANCED: An effective format regardless of fitness level, *The One-Minute Workout* program (fully outlined on page 9) prescribes the use of resistance exercises for one-minute intervals to develop 10 major muscle groups:

1. Back
2. Chest
3. Shoulders
4. Triceps
5. Biceps
6. Quadriceps/Buttocks
7. Hamstrings
8. Inner/Outer Thighs
9. Calves
10. Abs/Core

Developing your muscles helps to improve your metabolism, the processes that turn the food you eat into energy your body can use, and to increase your metabolic rate, the rate at which your body burns calories and fat. The higher the percentage of muscle your body carries, the higher the percentage of fat your body burns, even at rest.

As you work out, keep in mind these *Basic Resistance Training Tips:*

1. Lift weight you can handle. Or use the supervision of a spotter/partner.
2. Don't unnecessarily rock or swing the weight too much during lifts.
3. Protect your spine (keep it flat, erect or slightly arched when appropriate).
4. Use proper form/technique.
5. Keep your feet firmly planted on the floor, footrests or foot-pads.
6. "Think with the muscle." (Flex or squeeze muscles with every contraction).
7. Hydrate! Constantly replenish the water you lose through sweat.
8. Fight through the "desire to quit" to increase your body-reshaping potential.
9. Breath! Exhale during the contraction or exertion part of each movement and inhale during the extension or relaxation part of the movement.
10. Follow safety instructions on exercise machines or consult a fitness trainer.

Refer to the list of *Resistance Training Exercises* (page 53) complete with demonstrations and descriptions.

NOVICE, INTERMEDIATE and ADVANCED: For all fitness levels, the *One-Minute Workout* program recommends the use of cardiovascular/aerobic exercises in conjunction with your resistance training exercises.

As you work out, keep in mind these *Basic Cardiovascular/Aerobic Training Tips:*

1. Aim for no less than 20 minutes of vigorous cardiovascular activity daily.
2. Protect your spine (keep it flat, erect or slightly arched when appropriate).
3. Use proper form/technique.
4. Hydrate! Replenish the water you lose through sweat.
5. Breath! Constantly inhale and exhale to aid in your endurance.
6. Endure! Complete your workouts to increase your fat-burning potential.
7. Cushion the impact on your joints by landing properly on your heels, toes or planted feet when running, jogging, leaping or jumping.
8. Follow safety instructions on cardio equipment or consult a fitness trainer.

Refer to the list of *Cardiovascular/Aerobic Exercises* (pages 88–89) Select the one you enjoy most.

DRILL 4 • Work Through It!

NOVICE, INTERMEDIATE and ADVANCED: There is a heavy mental component to all of this talk about the body. Use your mind not just your muscles to get through your workouts. Workouts should challenge you, and will require mental, as well as physical, strength to complete.

Of course, if you experience severe pain or discomfort, i.e., pain that makes it difficult for you to continue exercising, stop and consult a physician.

However, don't confuse mild soreness or burning muscles as a signal to stop exercising. You may feel a slight "burn"—it's your body reacting to the exercise. In response, your tested muscles will repair themselves and get leaner and stronger to better handle your next workout.

When you feel as though you want to quit before you've completed the last repetition of an exercise set or the last few minutes of a cardio session, your mental power must kick in and challenge you to work through the perceived barrier and finish it. That is the point when your body changes. That's how you see results.

DRILL 5 • Wind Down!

NOVICE, INTERMEDIATE and ADVANCED: After you complete an exercise session, cool down with stretches (pages 47–52). Light, properly executed stretches relax the muscles to minimize post-workout soreness, and this gives you a chance to mentally debrief the day's activities.

Refer to the list of *Stretching Exercises* complete with demonstrations and descriptions. Perform lower body stretches after training your lower body. Perform upper body stretches after training your upper body.

Real Deal Training Principles

Repair/rejuvenate your body with rest.
Elevate your metabolic rate with cardio exercise.
Activate your muscles with resistance training.
Loosen/lengthen your body with stretching exercises.

DRILL 6 • **Work Your Way Up!**

NOVICE, INTERMEDIATE and ADVANCED: After you achieve your first goal to get started on a regular workout program, make "progress" your second goal. Work your way up when your body says you are ready to graduate. If you start lifting five pounds, eventually work up to lifting seven and then ten pounds. If you start doing 20 minutes of cardio, eventually work up to doing 30 and then 45 minutes.

Use *The REAL DEAL Personal Log* (page 91) to keep track of your ongoing goals and personal progress toward an overall healthier lifestyle. Continue to challenge yourself and take your fitness to the next level. Over time, you'll progress from Novice level to Intermediate level to Advanced level. In turn, you can look back on your success and marvel at how a simple *One-Minute Workout* program contributed to a lifetime of healthy joy.

In conclusion, we break down the acronym R.E.A.L. as a handy reminder of basic principles to keep in mind as you plan your training program. They represent a summery of what has been covered so far in *The REAL DEAL Training Guide*.

Next, we will examine the foundation upon which this manual is built: *The One-Minute Workout* program—a simple program in which everyone can participate and excel.

Real Deal Training Principles
Remember to have fun. Results are on the other side of the hard work.
Expect mild post-workout soreness- it's your body changing, which isn't easy.
Acquaint yourself with your goals. Log them, along with the actions you take.
Learn to appreciate sweat. It's the byproduct of hard work. The more, the better.

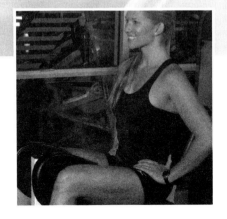

CHAPTER 3
THE ONE-MINUTE WORKOUT PROGRAM

The One-Minute Workout program is effective regardless of your fitness level, from the **Novice** exerciser with little to no history of physical activity to the **Intermediate** exerciser currently engaged in physical activity. The **Advanced** exerciser maintaining a healthy and physically active lifestyle can adjust the program to meet his or her needs as well.

The One-Minute Workout program is a simple program based on a one-minute principle: train each major muscle group with one minute of moderate resistance exercise split by one-minute aerobic intervals.

Let's combine resistance training exercises (pages 53–87) and the options for cardiovascular/aerobic exercises (pages 88–89), and design a *One-Minute Workout* program for you. Select your fitness level (**Novice**, **Intermediate**, or **Advanced**) and start to sweat.

In addition, we have included pre-designed, theme-based *One-Minute Workout* programs you can choose to use immediately (pages 16–19).

FITNESS LEVEL 1 • **Novice**

Exercise Experience: Little to none

Program Duration: Approximately 4-8 Weeks (Then proceed to Intermediate)

Days Per Week: 2 Days

Workout Plan: 1 *One-Minute Workout* Session

1 Cardio Workout Session

DAY 1 • One-Minute Workout

Use lightweight (not heavy) resistance or just body weight. Perform one resistance exercise (see pages 53–87) per muscle group listed below for one minute. (Total Time: 10 Minutes)

1. Back
2. Chest
3. Shoulders
4. Triceps
5. Biceps
6. Quadriceps/Buttocks
7. Hamstrings
8. Inner/Outer Thighs
9. Calves
10. Abs/Core

Example		
Target	**Exercises**	**Duration**
Back	Bent-over Rows	1 minute
Chest	Pushups	1 minute
Shoulders	Shoulder Press	1 minute
Triceps	Dips	1 minute
Biceps	Dumbbell Curls	1 minute
Quads	Squats	1 minute
Hamstrings	Deadlifts	1 minute
Outer Thigh	Karate Kicks	1 minute
Calves	Calf Raises	1 minute
Abs	Crunches	1 minute

DAY 2 • 20-Minute Cardio Workout

Select an exercise from the list of cardiovascular/aerobic exercises (see pages 88–89). Perform one activity or multiple indoor activities for 20 minutes or participate in an outdoor sport/activity for 20 minutes.

NOTE: Repeat Day 1 Workout and Day 2 Workout with a day of rest in between for 4 to 8 weeks.

Example	
Novice Workout Plan: January and February	
Monday:	Day 1 One-Minute Workout
Tuesday:	Rest/Day off
Wednesday:	Day 2: Cardio Workout

After 4 to 8 weeks, proceed to Intermediate level workouts (pages 11–12).

FITNESS LEVEL 2 • Intermediate*

Exercise Experience: Exercising for 6 or more months

Program Duration: Approximately 6-12 Weeks (Then proceed to Advanced)

Days Per Week: 3 Days

Workout Plan: 1 One-Minute Workout Session

1 Upper-Body Workout Session & Cardio Workout

1 Lower-Body Workout Session & Cardio Workout

DAY 1 • One-Minute Workout

Use moderate resistance (slightly increased from Novice level and based on your newly gained strength—if you were using 5-pound dumbbells before, use 10-pound weights now). Perform one resistance exercise (see pages 53–87) per muscle group for one minute. Split each group with a one-minute aerobic interval. (Total Time: 20 Minutes)

1. Back
2. Chest
3. Shoulders
4. Triceps
5. Biceps
6. Quadriceps/Buttocks
7. Hamstrings
8. Inner/Outer Thighs
9. Calves
10. Abs/Core

---

* These are suggested programs. Adjust to fit your specific level of skill, strength or endurance or to suit your specific fitness goals by simply increasing the resistance level, duration or intensity.

Example

Target	Exercises	Duration
Back	Bent-over Rows	1 minute
Cardio:	*Jogging in place*	*1 minute*
Chest	Pushups	1 minute
Cardio:	*Jumping Jacks*	*1 minute*
Shoulders	Shoulder Press	1 minute
Cardio:	*Jogging in place*	*1 minute*
Triceps	Dips	1 minute
Cardio:	*Jumping Jacks*	*1 minute*
Biceps	Dumbbell Curls	1 minute
Cardio:	*Jogging in place*	*1 minute*
Quads	Squats	1 minute
Cardio:	*Jumping Jacks*	*1 minute*
Hamstrings	Deadlifts	1 minute
Cardio:	*Jogging in place*	*1 minute*
Outer Thigh	Karate Kicks	1 minute
Cardio:	*Jumping Jacks*	*1 minute*
Calves	Calf Raises	1 minute
Cardio:	*Jogging in place*	*1 minute*
Abs	Crunches	1 minute
Cardio:	*Jumping Jacks*	*1 minute*

DAY 2 • Upper-Body Resistance Training Workout

Plus *20-Minute Cardio Workout*

Use moderate resistance (weight you can handle but also presents a challenge—if you easily lift 5 pounds but can't lift 10 pounds, use 7-pound weights). Perform two upper-body resistance exercises (see pages 53–70) per muscle group for three sets of 12–15 repetitions each. (Total Time: Approximately 30 Minutes)

Example

Muscle Group	Exercises	Sets x Reps
Back	Pick 2	3 x 12 to 15
Chest	Pick 2	3 x 12 to 15
Shoulders	Pick 2	3 x 12 to 15
Biceps	Pick 2	3 x 12 to 15
Triceps	Pick 2	3 x 12 to 15
Abs/Core	Pick 2	3 x 12 to 15

Follow (or precede) this with a 20-minute session of the cardiovascular/aerobic exercise of your choice (see pages 88–89).

DAY 3 • Lower-Body Resistance Training Workout

Plus *20-Minute Cardio Workout*

Use moderate resistance (weight you can handle but also presents a challenge—if you easily push 40 pounds but can't push 60 pounds, use 50 pounds). Perform two lower-body resistance exercises (see pages 71–81) per muscle group for three sets of 12 to 15 repetitions each. (Total Time: Approximately 30 Minutes)

Example

Muscle Group	Exercises	Sets x Reps
Quadriceps/Butt	Pick 2	3 x 12 to 15
Hamstrings	Pick 2	3 x 12 to 15
Inner/Outer Thighs	Pick 2	3 x 12 to 15
Calves	Pick 2	3 x 12 to 15
Abs/Core	Pick 2	3 x 12 to 15

Follow (or precede) this with a 20-minute session of the cardiovascular/aerobic exercise of your choice (see pages 88–89).

NOTE: Repeat Day 1 Workout, Day 2 Workout and Day 3 Workout with at least one day of rest in between each workout for 6 to 12 weeks.

Example

Intermediate Workout Plan: March, April and May

Monday:	Day 1 One-Minute Workout
Tuesday:	Rest/Day off
Wednesday:	Day 2: Upper-Body Workout plus Cardio
Thursday:	Rest/Day off
Friday:	Day 3: Lower-Body Workout plus Cardio

After 6 to 12 weeks, proceed to Advanced level workouts (pages 13–15).

FITNESS LEVEL 3 • Advanced*

Exercise Experience: Exercising 12 or more months

Program Duration: Approximately 12 Weeks and beyond

Days Per Week: 4 Days

Workout Plan: 1 *One-Minute Workout* Session

1 Upper-Body Workout Session & Cardio Workout

1 Lower-Body Workout Session & Cardio Workout

1 Workout of Your Choice

DAY 1 • One-Minute Workout

Use moderate resistance (slightly increased from Intermediate level and based on your newly gained strength—if you were using 10-pound dumbbells before, use 15-pound weights now). Perform two resistance exercises (see pages 53–87) per muscle group for one minute. Split each muscle groups' two exercises with a one-minute aerobic interval. (Total Time: 30 Minutes)

1. Back
2. Chest
3. Shoulders
4. Triceps
5. Biceps
6. Quadriceps/Buttocks
7. Hamstrings
8. Inner/Outer Thighs
9. Calves
10. Abs/Core

---

* These are suggested programs. Adjust to fit your specific level of skill, strength or endurance or to suit your specific fitness goals by simply increasing the resistance level, duration or intensity.

Example

Target	Exercises	Duration
Back	Bent-over Rows	1 minute
Cardio:	*Jogging in place*	*1 minute*
Back	Pulldowns	1 minute
Chest	Pushups	1 minute
Cardio:	*Jumping Jacks*	*1 minute*
Chest	Incline Press	1 minute
Shoulders	Shoulder Press	1 minute
Cardio:	*Jogging in place*	*1 minute*
Shoulders	Lateral Raises	1 minute
Triceps	Dips	1 minute
Cardio:	*Jumping Jacks*	*1 minute*
Triceps	Pushdowns	1 minute
Biceps	Dumbbell Curls	1 minute
Cardio:	*Jogging in place*	*1 minute*
Biceps	Barbell Curls	1 minute
Quads	Squats	1 minute
Cardio:	*Jumping Jacks*	*1 minute*
Quads	Lunges	1 minute
Hamstrings	Deadlifts	1 minute
Cardio:	*Jogging in place*	*1 minute*
Hamstrings	Lying Leg Curl	1 minute
Outer Thigh	Karate Kicks	1 minute
Cardio:	*Jumping Jacks*	*1 minute*

Target	Exercises	Duration
Inner Thigh	Adductor	1 minute
Calves	Seated Calf Raises	1 minute
Cardio:	*Jogging in place*	*1 minute*
Calves	Standing Calf Raises	1 minute
Abs	Crunches	1 minute
Cardio:	*Jumping Jacks*	*1 minute*
Abs	Oblique Twists	1 minute

DAY 2 • Upper-Body Resistance Training Workout

Plus *20- to 30-Minute Cardio Workout*

Use moderate resistance (weight you can handle but also presents a challenge—if you easily lift 5 pounds but can't lift 10 pounds, use 7-pound weights). Perform two upper-body resistance exercises (see pages 53–70) per muscle group for three sets of 15 repetitions each. (Total Time: Approximately 45 Minutes)

Example		
Muscle Group	**Exercises**	**Sets x Reps**
Back	Pick 2	3 x 15
Chest	Pick 2	3 x 15
Shoulders	Pick 2	3 x 15
Biceps	Pick 2	3 x 15
Triceps	Pick 2	3 x 15
Abs/Core	Pick 2	3 x 15

Follow (or precede) this with 20 to 30 minutes of the cardiovascular/aerobic exercise (see pages 88–89) of your choice.

DAY 3 • Lower-Body Resistance Training Workout

Plus *20- to 30-Minute Cardio Workout*

Use moderate resistance (weight you can handle but also presents a challenge—if you easily push 40 pounds but can't push 60 pounds, use 50 pounds). Perform two lower-body resistance exercises (see pages 71–81) per muscle group listed below for three sets of 15 repetitions each. (Total Time: Approximately 45 Minutes)

Example		
Muscle Group	**Exercises**	**Sets x Reps**
Quadriceps/Butt	Pick 2	3 x 15
Hamstrings	Pick 2	3 x 15
Inner/Outer Thighs	Pick 2	3 x 15
Calves	Pick 2	3 x 15
Abs/Core	Pick 2	3 x 15

Follow (or precede) this with 20 to 30 minutes of the cardiovascular/aerobic exercise of your choice (see pages 88–89).

DAY 4 • 45-Minute Cardio Workout

OR *Repeat Day 1*

OR *Repeat Day 2 (selecting different upper-body exercises)*

Choose among the following options for your fourth workout day of the week:

Perform a 45-minute session of the cardiovascular/aerobic exercise of your choice (see pages 88–89).

Repeat *One-Minute Workout*

Perform anther Upper-Body Workout (with different exercises)

NOTE: Repeat Workouts from Day 1, Day 2, Day 3 and Day 4 with at least one day of rest in between each workout on an ongoing basis.

Example

Advanced Workout Plan: July and going forward

Monday:	Day 1 One-Minute Workout
Tuesday:	Rest/Day off
Wednesday:	Day 2: Upper-Body Workout plus Cardio
Thursday:	Rest/Day off
Friday:	Day 3: Lower-Body Workout plus Cardio
Saturday:	Rest/Day off
Sunday:	Day 4: Workout of your choice
Monday:	Rest/Day off
Tuesday:	Day 1 One-Minute Workout

And so on following this pattern…

After 12 weeks, continue to follow the pattern above evermore, with the variety necessary to stay motivated. It's now a lifestyle.

SAMPLE ONE-MINUTE WORKOUT PROGRAMS

You have been introduced to *The One-Minute Workout*. If you need ideas for how to organize your program, below are four pre-designed *One-Minute Workout* Programs from which you can choose.

Feel free to rotate these routines. Perform one resistance exercise per muscle group for one minute. Refer to the exercise demonstrations (pages 53–87) for full descriptions (as well as other exercises that can be substituted to suit individual tastes or abilities). Split these exercise with one-minute intervals of cardiovascular/aerobic exercises (pages 88–89).

ONE-MINUTE WORKOUT 1

THE PUSH/PULL WORKOUT

Target	Exercises	Duration
Back	Pulldowns or Pull-Ups	1 minute
Cardio:	*Jumping Jacks*	*1 minute*
Chest	Pushups	1 minute
Cardio:	*Jogging in Place*	*1 minute*
Shoulders	Lateral Deltoid Raises	1 minute
Cardio:	*Squat Thrusts*	*1 minute*
Triceps	Bench Dips	1 minute
Cardio:	*Side-to-Side Shuffling*	*1 minute*
Biceps	Concentration Curls	1 minute
Cardio:	*Jumping Lunges*	*1 minute*

Target	Exercises	Duration
Quads	Step-Ups	1 minute
Cardio:	*Jumping Jacks*	*1 minute*
Hamstrings	Leg Curls (Standing)	1 minute
Cardio:	*Jogging in Place*	*1 minute*
Inner/Outer Thighs	Adductor/Abductor	1 minute
Cardio:	*Squat Thrusts*	*1 minute*
Calves	Single-Leg Standing Calf Raises	1 minute
Cardio:	*Side-to-Side Shuffling*	*1 minute*
Abs	Crunches (Legs Elevated)	1 minute
Cardio:	*Jumping Lunges*	*1 minute*

ONE-MINUTE WORKOUT 2

THE BARBELL WORKOUT

Target	Exercises	Duration
Back	Bent-Over Rows (Barbell)	1 minute
Cardio:	*Jumping Jacks*	*1 minute*
Chest	Flat Chest Presses (Barbell)	1 minute
Cardio:	*Jogging in Place*	*1 minute*
Shoulders	Shoulder Presses (Barbell)	1 minute
Cardio:	*Squat Thrusts*	*1 minute*
Triceps	Lying Triceps Extensions (Barbell)	1 minute
Cardio:	*Side-to-Side Shuffling*	*1 minute*
Biceps	Barbell Curls	1 minute
Cardio:	*Jumping Lunges*	*1 minute*
Quads	Squats (Barbell)	1 minute
Cardio:	*Jumping Jacks*	*1 minute*
Hamstrings (Barbell)	Stiff-Legged Deadlifts	1 minute
Cardio:	*Jogging in Place*	*1 minute*
Inner/Outer Thighs	Wide-Stance Side-to-Side Squat (Barbell)	1 minute
Cardio:	*Squat Thrusts*	*1 minute*
Calves (Barbell)	Standing Calf Raises	1 minute
Cardio:	*Side-to-Side Shuffling*	*1 minute*
Abs	Reverse (Low-Ab) Crunches	1 minute
Cardio:	*Jumping Lunges*	*1 minute*

ONE-MINUTE WORKOUT 3

THE DOUBLE-DUMBBELL WORKOUT

Target	Exercises	Duration
Back	Bent-Over Rows (Dumbbells)	1 minute
Cardio:	*Jumping Jacks*	*1 minute*
Chest	Flat Chest Flyes	1 minute
Cardio:	*Jogging in Place*	*1 minute*
Shoulders	Front Deltoid Raises	1 minute
Cardio:	*Squat Thrusts*	*1 minute*
Triceps	Triceps Kickbacks	1 minute
Cardio:	*Side-to-Side Shuffling*	*1 minute*
Biceps	Dumbbell Curls	1 minute
Cardio:	*Jumping Lunges*	*1 minute*
Quads	Lunges (with Dumbbells)	1 minute
Cardio:	*Jumping Jacks*	*1 minute*

Target	Exercises	Duration
Hamstrings	Stiff-Legged Deadlifts (Dumbbells)	1 minute
Cardio:	*Jogging in Place*	*1 minute*
Inner/Outer Thighs	Adductor/Abductor (Lying on side, hold dumbbell against leg)	1 minute
Cardio:	*Squat Thrusts*	*1 minute*
Calves (Dumbbells)	Standing Calf Raises	1 minute
Cardio:	*Side-to-Side Shuffling*	*1 minute*
Abs	Crunches (Hold dumbbell behind neck)	1 minute
Cardio:	*Jumping Lunges*	*1 minute*

ONE-MINUTE WORKOUT 4

THE MACHINE WORKOUT

Target	Exercises	Duration
Back	Seated Rows (cable row machine)	1 minute
Cardio:	*Jumping Jacks*	*1 minute*
Chest	Cable Crossover	1 minute
Cardio:	*Jogging in Place*	*1 minute*
Shoulders	Rear Deltoid Machine	1 minute
Cardio:	*Squat Thrusts*	*1 minute*
Triceps	Triceps Pushdowns	1 minute
Cardio:	*Side-to-Side Shuffling*	*1 minute*
Biceps	Biceps Curl Machine	1 minute
Cardio:	*Jumping Lunges*	*1 minute*

Target	Exercises	Duration
Quads	Leg Presses	1 minute
Cardio:	*Jumping Jacks*	*1 minute*
Hamstrings	Leg Curls (Lying or Seated)	1 minute
Cardio:	*Jogging in Place*	*1 minute*
Inner/Outer Thighs	Adductor/Abductor Machines	1 minute
Cardio:	*Squat Thrusts*	*1 minute*
Calves	Standing Calf Raises (Dumbbells)	1 minute
Cardio:	*Side-to-Side Shuffling*	*1 minute*
Abs	Abs Crunch Machine	1 minute
Cardio:	*Jumping Lunges*	*1 minute*

REAL DEAL NUTRITION
THE EATING GUIDE

WELCOME TO REAL DEAL EATING

We tackled the importance of training and exercise in *The REAL DEAL Training Guide*; now, let's address the second, and equally critical, component of your tool kit: eating and nutrition. Welcome to REAL DEAL Eating.

Healthy eating means engaging in habits and practices that contribute to proper nutrition and good health. *The REAL DEAL Eating Guide* includes tips and recommendations focused on a balance of variety, supplementation and portion control.

The guide is structured around *The REAL DEAL Dietary Guidelines*—seven simple rules for healthy eating.

Rule 1 is about food variety and references the Food Pyramid as a way to achieve a good meal mix. Rule 2 deals with carb consumption and points to the Glycemic Index as a way to check your food's carb content. Rule 3 concerns fat intake and compares "good cholesterol" to "bad cholesterol." Rule 4 covers calorie burning and suggests weight-management tips. Rule 5 addresses alcohol consumption and breaks down serving sizes. Rule 6 looks at sugar and describes the sugar content in certain foods. Rule 7 pertains to salt intake and lists foods that can help counteract the effects of too much sodium.

The section for each rule closes with *REAL DEAL Nutrition Principles*. These principles sum up the main points and are handy little reminders for how to apply each rule to your eating habits.

We finish off with *The REAL DEAL Meal Plan*, an easy-to-follow program designed to help you map out your meals. Dig in and enjoy.

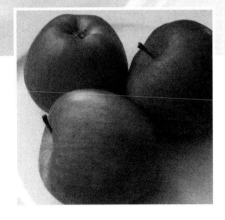

CHAPTER 4
THE REAL DEAL DIETARY GUIDELINES

Based on the United States Department of Agriculture's recommended dietary guidelines (*www.usda.gov*), following are *The REAL DEAL Dietary Guidelines*:

Rule 1: Mix It Up!
Rule 2: Get Carb Smart!
Rule 3: Avoid Bad Fat!
Rule 4: Burn Your Food!
Rule 5: Limit Your Booze!
Rule 6: Skip The Sugar!
Rule 7: Shake The Salt!

Let's explore these Rules and provide R.E.A.L. Principles to help you put each one into practice. Use *The REAL DEAL Eating Log* included in this guidebook (page 102) to keep track of your objectives and achievements.

RULE 1 • Mix It Up!

Eat a variety of foods, since no single food supplies all the nutrients in the amounts you need for good health. Consume the United States Department of Agriculture's recommended number of servings daily from each of the five major food groups based on the Food Pyramid:

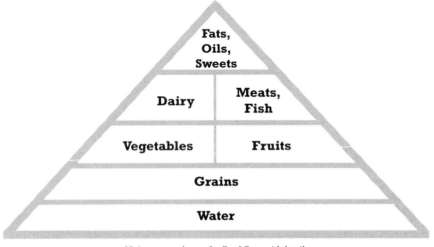

Visit www.usda.org for Food Pyramid details.

FOOD PYRAMID

Consume more daily servings from each group as you descend the pyramid.

- Fats, Oils, Sweets Sparingly
- Dairy 2-4 Servings
- Meats/Fish 2-3 Servings
- Vegetables 3-5 Servings
- Fruits 4-6 Servings
- Grains 6-11 Servings
- Water 8 Servings

When mixing up your meals, it's helpful to know which foods to eat more of and which foods to consume less. See page 95 for the *More or Less List,* a handy guide for what to partake in and what to pass on. Also, the Nutrition Facts labels on food packages can assist you in making informed choices about how the combination of foods you select contribute to a varied, healthy nutrition program. See page 96 for tips on how to read and use the information on Nutrition Facts labels. Also, be sure to pair your mix of food with plenty of water.

REAL DEAL Nutrition Principles (for Variety)

Read Nutrition Facts labels on food packages to track caloric & nutrient intake.

Eat low-fat or fat-free dairy products for sufficient calcium without the excess fat.

Ask your doctor if you need nutritional supplements for special health needs.

Lean toward unrefined foods for the nutrients your body needs for good health.

Water is second only to oxygen as essential for life. Many people don't drink enough water and, in turn, suffer from dehydration. The primary reason for sufficient water intake is to replenish the large percentage of water that comprises the human body. Because two thirds of our body weight is water (40 to 50 quarts), we must replace 2.5 quarts of water every day. We are water. So we need a lot of it to stay healthy and carry out our bodies' functions. Water cushions and protects joints, tissues and organs, carries nutrients and oxygen to cells, regulates body temperature and blood circulation, helps with digestion and food absorption, and removes toxins and wastes. Avoid dehydration. If your body tries to operate with insufficient water, it reacts with symptoms, illnesses, and/or diseases. So consume 6 to 8 glasses of water per day.

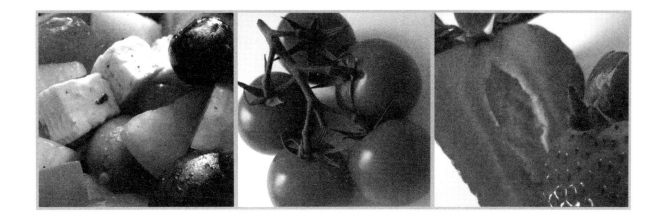

RULE 2 • Get Carb Smart!

Carbohydrates are the human body's main energy source. The two main types are simple carbs (or "simple sugars") and complex carbs (or "complex sugars"). Carbs are classified into sugars, starches and dietary fiber. Generally, sugars are "simple carbs," and starches and fiber are "complex carbs." However, fructose (fruit sugar) is a simple carb that behaves like a complex carb. Complex carbs improve your digestion, stabilize the blood sugar, keep your energy at an even level, and help you feel satisfied longer after your meal.

In recent years, carbs have developed a bad reputation among promoters of commercially driven diet or weight-loss products. However, from a nutritional viewpoint, carbs are essential to any healthy eating program as they are rich sources of a range of vitamins, minerals, phyto-chemicals and other micronutrients. Low-carb diets are typically lacking in sufficient nutrition, which is why they often advise low-carb dieters to take multi-nutrient supplements.

FIBER IN GRAMS— EAT 20 TO 30 GRAMS DAILY

7.0 g 1 cup 40% bran cereal
7.0 g Half cup pinto beans
4.0 g Half cup split peas
4.0 g Half cup raisins
4.0 g 1 pear
3.0 g Half cup corn or peas
3.0 g Half cup cooked oatmeal
3.0 g 1 apple or orange
2.0 g 1 slice whole-wheat bread
1.0 g 1 cup popcorn
1.0 g Half cup celery or green beans
0.4 g 1 slice white bread
0.0 g animal-based foods have no fiber, these include meat, fish, poultry, cheese, eggs and milk

So, carbs are good if you get them from smart places, like grains, vegetables and fruits. What you want to watch out for are carbs that are more refined or "processed," such as table sugar and white-flour foods. "Refined" simple carbs (usually the "sweet stuff") are classified as such because nutrients required for the metabolism of the contained sugar are removed during the refining process. Without those nutrients, your body pulls stored nutrients to metabolize the sugar. When those nutrient stores are overworked, your weakened body is vulnerable to sickness.

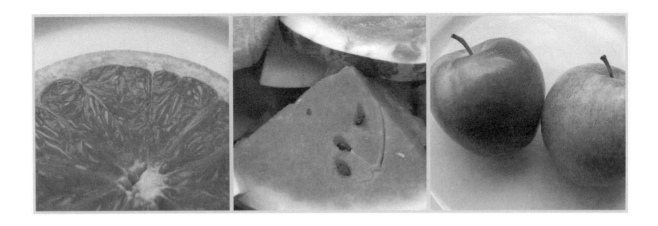

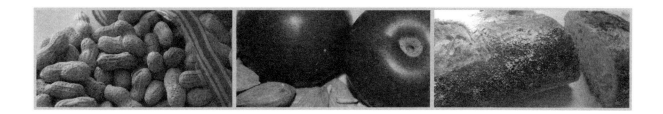

Most refining processes remove nearly all fiber, which slows the release of the sugar into the system. The fiber in fruits—which are unrefined simple carbs—helps make the sugar in fruit so much healthier than the sugar in refined carbohydrates. That's why drinking concentrated, processed fruit juice, doesn't provide the same healthy benefits as eating whole fruit. The latter retains the natural fiber and decreases your sugar intake, while the sugars consumed are less concentrated.

The Glycemic Index (page 98) divides carbohydrate-containing foods into high-, medium- or low-glycemic index foods. Weight-loss plans based on the glycemic index (GI), which classifies carbs according to their effect on blood glucose after digestion (i.e., how fast they are digested, and, thus, how quickly they raise blood sugar levels), offer all the metabolic health benefits of so-called low-carb diets, without any of the nutritional concerns of long-term carb restriction. Failure to maintain blood sugar leads to high (hyperglycemia) or low (hypoglycemia) blood sugar. High blood sugar, frequent hunger. Low blood sugar, low energy.

REAL DEAL Nutrition Principles (for Carbs)

Rack up most of the calories in your diet from wholegrains, veggies and fruits.

Eat adequate fiber for proper bowel functioning & reduction in diverticular disease (ruptured colon).

Aim for complex carbs prepared or served in their low-calorie state.

Lower your risk for chronic diseases (like heart disease & cancers) with smart carbs.

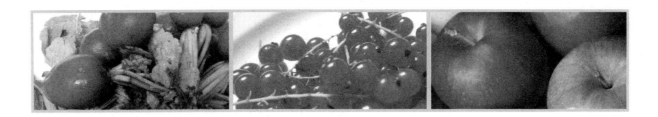

RULE 3 • Avoid Bad Fat!

Fats are concentrated sources of calories. There are three main types of fats in food: **Saturated Fat** (in red meats and red meat products, such as pork, beef and lamb and in dairy products; in tropical oils such as palm oil, palm kernel oil, and coconut oil; and in vegetables oils chemically altered to form a solid at room temperature—i.e., Trans-Fats); **Monounsaturated Fats** (in plant oils such as olive, peanut, and canola oil; liquid at room temperature but solidify when cooled); **Polyunsaturated Fats** (in plant oils such as corn, sunflower, safflower or soybean oil; in fish as omega-3 fat, which may help protect against heart disease by slowing blood clotting; remain liquid even at cold temperatures).

You need some fats, because they supply energy and essential fatty acids and they promote absorption of the fat-soluble vitamins A, D, E and K. However, saturated fat is the most harmful. Because high levels of saturated fat and cholesterol in the diet are linked to increased blood cholesterol (page 99), as well as greater risk of heart disease. When you eat too much saturated fat, your body reacts by making more cholesterol than it needs, and the surplus ends up in your blood.

Monounsaturated and polyunsaturated fats help lower blood cholesterol levels by helping your body get rid of newly formed cholesterol. So these fats should replace (not accompany) some of the saturated fat in your eating plan. Basically, fat contains nine calories per gram, whereas protein and carbohydrates only contain four calories per gram. So, using a large amount of monounsaturated or polyunsaturated fats to lower cholesterol will backfire, because the extra calories will make you gain weight, which will push up your cholesterol levels.

Only animal foods contain cholesterol—plant foods do not contain cholesterol. In animals, as in humans, cholesterol is a part of all cells and serves many vital functions. Therefore, foods of animal origin—such as meat, poultry, fish, eggs, or milk—all contain some cholesterol. Generally, foods high in animal fat are also high in cholesterol. Two exceptions are liver and egg yolks, which are *not* high in fat but *are* high in cholesterol. See page 99 for a comparison between "good" cholesterol and "bad" cholesterol.

REAL DEAL Nutrition Principles (for Fats)

Reduce cholesterol by cooking with light vegetable oils versus more fatty oils.

Estimate fat intake based on weight-loss goals (20-30% of total calories is ideal).

Avoid animal fats, which are high in saturated fat and cholesterol.

Limit daily intake of saturated fat to no more than 5% to 7% of total calories.

RULE 4 • Burn Your Food!

You must maintain a healthy body weight. The way to do this is to burn off the calories you consume through food, which serves as your body's fuel, with daily exercise. Start with the workout programs in *The REAL DEAL Training Guide* (page 3). Weight gain increases your risk for high blood pressure, heart disease, stroke, diabetes, cancers, arthritis, breathing problems and other illness.

REAL DEAL Nutrition Principles (for Burning Calories)

Refuel with healthy portions of food to perform exercise & daily activities.

Engage in more vigorous activity to help reduce body fat and disease risk.

Aim for no less than 20 to 30 minutes of moderate physical activity every day.

Lessen the time involved in sedentary activities (sitting) that burn no calories.

RULE 5 • Limit Your Booze!

Alcohol is not recommended at all; however, if you choose to drink, drink in moderation. Alcoholic beverages supply calories but few to no nutrients.

ONE DRINK IS EQUAL TO:
- one 12-ounce can of beer
- one 5-ounce glass of wine
- one 1.5-ounce shot of liquor

DON'T DARE DRINK IF YOU:
- Are Underage
- Are pregnant or trying to conceive
- Cannot restrict drinking to moderate levels
- Use prescription or over-the-counter medications
- Plan to drive or participate in activities that require attention or skill

REAL DEAL Nutrition Principles (for Alcohol)

Reduce high blood pressure, stroke, heart disease & cancer risk by forgoing alcohol.

Eliminate, if possible, alcohol when you are on a low-calorie, weight-loss program.

Avoid chronic alcoholic use to prevent dependency, impaired judgment or accidents.

Limit alcohol to one drink per day for women or two drinks per day for men.

RULE 6 • Skip The Sugar!

Sugars added to sweeten foods supply calories but few or no nutrients. Consume sugars in moderation. According to USDA surveys, the average American consumes 20 teaspoons of added sugar (sugar not naturally found in milk and fruit) each day, which is double the USDA's recommendation of no more than 10 teaspoons of added sugar per day.

SUGAR INTAKE ADDS UP QUICKLY

- A 12-ounce soda contains 10 teaspoons of sugar
- An 8-ounce lemonade contains about 7 teaspoons of sugar
- A 2-ounce package of candy contains 11 teaspoons of sugar
- A cup of frosted cereal contains more than 4 teaspoons of sugar

Alternatives to refined sugar include brand name non-caloric sweeteners and Stevia (an herb with therapeutic properties). In addition, fruit can often be used as a natural replacement for sugar, for example raisins or dates to sweeten baked goods, bananas on cereal, or pure fruit juice to replace soft drinks.

REAL DEAL Nutrition Principles (for Sugars)

Ration all sugars: table sugar, molasses, honey, syrup, sucrose, and fructose.

Eliminate sugar, when possible, if you have weight-loss or low-calorie needs.

Assess sugar content per serving by consulting labels (1 teaspoon is 4 grams).

Limit intake of sugar beverages (soda, artificial juices, sweetened tea or coffee).

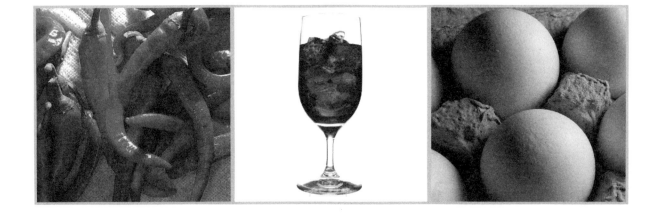

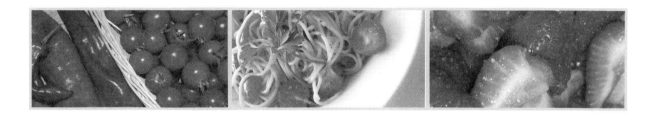

RULE 7 • Shake The Salt!

Small amounts of sodium and sodium chloride (salt) occur naturally in foods. Processed foods often contain higher levels of salt and sodium. Sodium plays an essential role in the regulation of fluids and blood pressure. High sodium intake is linked to hypertension (high blood pressure). Weight loss, physical activity, and increased potassium intake help to lower blood pressure.

Basically, blood pressure is a measure of the force of the blood pushing against the walls of your arteries. If it's high, your blood is pushing against the artery walls with too much pressure. According to the National Heart, Lung, and Blood Institute, a blood pressure level of 140/90 or higher is considered high. Between 120/80 and 139/89 mmHg signals pre-hypertension (a likelihood to develop high blood pressure if preventative measures are not taken); 120/80 is normal or ideal. High blood pressure has great consequences but few or no symptoms. The only sure way to find out if you have elevated blood pressure is to get checked by a healthcare professional.

Decreasing salt intake is advisable to reduce the risk of elevated blood pressure. Maintaining normal blood pressure reduces the risk of coronary heart disease, stroke, congestive heart failure, and kidney disease. Nutritional adjustments can prevent or delay the onset of high blood pressure and can lower elevated blood pressure. These lifestyles changes include reducing salt intake, increasing calcium and potassium intake and eating an overall healthful diet.

REAL DEAL Nutrition Principles (for Sodium)

Reduce intake of processed/packaged foods and eat more fresh fruits & veggies.

Elevate calcium and potassium intake, since high salt intake may increase calcium loss in the urine of salt eaters.

Avoid adding salt or salty sauces/condiments, as most food already contains salt.

Limit sodium to 2,300 mg per day (approximately 1 teaspoon of salt).

FOODS THAT ARE HIGH IN...

CALCIUM (in mg)
- **415 mg** 1 cup yogurt
- **300 mg** 1 cup skim milk
- **195 mg** 3 oz. canned salmon
- **160 mg** 1 cup broccoli
- **130 mg** 3½ oz. tofu
- **100 mg** Half cup collard greens
- **90 mg** 1 cup pinto beans

POTASSIUM (in mg)
- **626 mg** Half cup dried fruit
- **608 mg** 1 potato
- **446 mg** Half cup winter squash
- **451 mg** 1 banana
- **419 mg** Half cup cooked spinach
- **254 mg** 1 tomato
- **250 mg** 1 orange

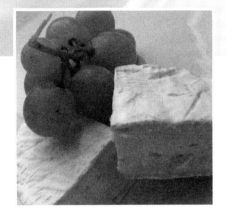

CHAPTER 5

THE REAL DEAL MEAL PLAN

THE REAL WAY TO EAT

Regulate portion size—servings should be no larger than the size of your palm.

Eat 5 to 6 small meals per day to help speed metabolism and burn body fat.

Avoid alcohol, foods high in saturated fat, sugar and excessive sodium (salt).

Load up on H2O—drink 8 to 10 glasses of water every day.

Breakdown of Daily Caloric Intake
Carbohydrates 55%-60%
Proteins 10%-20%
Fats less than 30%

REAL DEAL MEAL PLAN

Your meal planning will incorporate the following food blocks, which comprise the components of balanced eating.

FOOD BLOCK 1 • PROTEIN

What they are: Building Blocks

What they do: Help maintain and build muscle.

How to prepare: Broil, Grill, Bake or Steam

When to consume: Eat at each meal.

Examples: Chicken Breast, Chicken Salad, Turkey Breast, Lean Ground Turkey, Lean Ground Chicken, Lean Beef, Cod Fish, Tuna, Tuna Salad, Orange Roughy, Salmon, Scallops, Swordfish, Halibut, Tilapia, Lean Turkey Sausage, Lean Red Meat, Lean Pork, Egg Whites

FOOD BLOCK 2 • COMPLEX CARBS

What they are: Energy Fuel

What they do: Help energize and stimulate vitality.

How to prepare: Boil, Bake or Toast

When to consume: Eat in moderation early in the day.

Examples: Rice, Whole Wheat Breads, Pasta, Potatoes, Grits, Beans, Corn, Popcorn, Rice Cakes, Cereal (Bran, Fiber and Rice-based)

FOOD BLOCK 3 • FIBROUS CARBS

What they are: Fiber Source

What they do: Keep you full and provide essential vitamins.

How to prepare: Steam or Raw

When to consume: Eat any time.

Examples: Asparagus, Bean Sprouts, Broccoli, Cabbage, Collards/Turnips, Carrots (juice), Cauliflower, Celery, Cucumbers, Eggplant, Green Beans, Peas, Lettuce, Mushrooms, Onions, Peppers, Radishes, Scallions, Spinach, Squash, Tomatoes, Zucchini

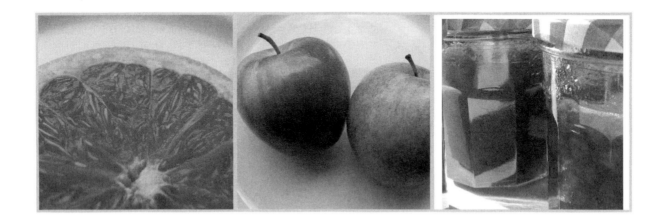

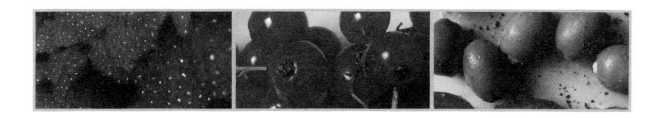

FOOD BLOCK 4 • SIMPLE CARBS

What they are: Energy Fuel

What they do: Keep you full and provide essential vitamins.

How to prepare: Fresh or Dry

When to consume: Eat any time. Good between-meal snacks.

Examples: Apple, Banana, Berries, Blueberries, Cantaloupe, Cranberries, Cherries, Grapefruit, Honeydew, Kiwi Fruit, Melons, Nectarine, Orange, Peach, Pineapple, Plum, Strawberries, Watermelon

FOOD BLOCK 5 • MEAL/PROTEIN SUPPLEMENTS

What they are: Pre- or Post-Workout Fuel

What they do: Supplement meals and provide essential vitamins.

How to prepare: N/A

When to consume: Once daily (multivitamins). Between-meal snacks (supplements).

Examples: Whey Protein (Bars, Drinks & Shakes), Flax Seed Oil, Omega 3, 6, 9 and Multivitamins. To supplement your daily food intake, take a multivitamin that contains ample amounts of the following vitamins and minerals: Vitamins A, B-6, B-12, C, D, E and K, Biotin, Calcium, Chloride, Chromium, Copper, Folic Acid, Iodine, Iron, Magnesium, Manganese, Molybdenum, Niacin, Pantothenic Acid, Phosphorus, Potassium, Riboflavin, Selenium and Zinc.

FOOD BLOCK 6 • MISCELLANEOUS

What they are: Extras, not Necessities

What they do: Add flavor.

How to prepare: N/A

When to consume: Consume sparingly.

Examples: Butter, Butter Substitute, Soy Milk, Ketchup, Lemon Juice, Margarine, Mustard, Nonfat Mayonnaise, Nonfat Salad Dressing, Salsa, Vinegar, Spices (Oregano, Garlic Powder, Onion Powder, Basil, Etc.)

AN IDEAL DAY ON THE REAL DEAL MEAL PLAN

Plan a five-meal day by consuming items from the food blocks. Select items from the block numbers represented and plug them into the equations below.

MEAL 1 (Breakfast):	1 + 2 + 3 or 5
MEAL 2 (Snack):	1 + 4 or 5
MEAL 3 (Lunch):	1 + 2 + 3 or 5
MEAL 4 (Snack):	1 + 3 + or 5
MEAL 5 (Dinner):	1 + 3 + 4 or 5
MEAL 6 (Snack):	1 + 3 + or 5 (optional)

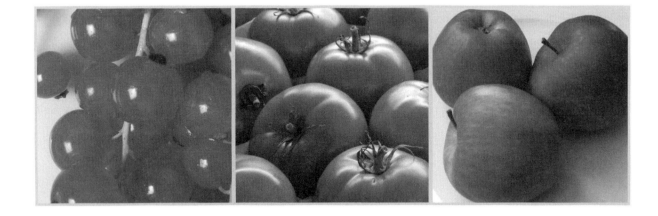

CHAPTER 6
REAL DEAL WELLNESS

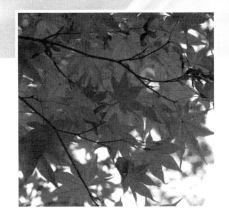

We have concentrated on fitness and focused on nutrition. Let's conclude by briefly touching upon the component of your tool kit that ties together all aspects of your health—lifestyle. Healthy living means engaging in habits and practices that contribute to overall wellness. Wellness is where your life inside and outside of the gym (training) and the kitchen (eating) co-mingle. It involves a balance of mind, body and soul, so we will provide you with motivational principles to help push you through the work you'll be doing on your fitness journey.

THE REAL TOTAL YOU

The three components of your total being are your mind, body and spirit/soul. Because it is virtually impossible to thrive without one of the three, try to develop each component with lifestyle routines.

THE MIND

Accountability focuses your mind and keeps you on the right path. This idea applies to other areas of your life such as finances and ethics, as well. How do you become financially responsible or morally responsible? You hold yourself or someone else holds you accountable for your actions. Similarly, maintenance of your fitness is ultimately up to you, but you may also have a doctor, trainer, workout partner or loved one who stays on top of you and checks you when you get off track. No, it's not always easy, but it's necessary. Everyone is capable of aspiring to be a healthier version of himself or herself. The way to stick to the plan is to know and understand that you're doing it for you. Love and respect yourself enough to commit to something that is good for you. If you give up on your health, the first and most important person that you will let down is you, followed by everyone who supports and loves you.

Address the mind through motivation and accountability. The following principles help improve your mental focus on your desired achievements and on your responsibility for your own success.

THE BODY

Your body needs proper rest and maintenance to thrive. They say, "Early to bed, early to rise makes us healthy, wealthy and wise." The wealthy part is debatable, but the healthy and wise parts hold true. It's wise, healthy and crucial to get the rest your body needs to recharge itself, particularly if you lead an active lifestyle. When you work your brain, heart and muscles all day, they need the hours of sleep to refresh and be ready to work the next day. Insufficient rest leaves your body and all of its systems functioning at low levels, which can dangerously affect your concentration at work, behind the wheel or during other tasks. Just remember, lots of sleep and rest do not translate into loafing or lying around excessively in lieu of doing other activities, especially exercise.

Even with adequate rest and physical activity, everyone is susceptible to disease. Exercise does not makes people exempt from regular checkups with a doctor. There are three ways to address health issues regardless of how you "feel":

REAL DEAL Wellness Principles—THE MIND

REAL Goals motivate us.

Recognize your potential and strive to achieve it by setting goals.
Estimate and evaluate the timetable for achieving your goals.
Allow yourself to bounce back from setbacks as you go for your goals.
Learn to reward yourself for goals achieved by setting new goals.

REAL Progress motivates us.

Reinforce your progress by tracking it with diaries, photos or milestones.
Earn success by progressing and achieving realistic, but aggressive, goals.
Accept that there is no progress without struggle and let that drive you.
Let mental toughness get you over the humps on the road to progress.

REAL Support motivates us.

Remain accountable by reporting to a workout partner, trainer or private journal.
Encourage those who encourage you to join in your healthy fitness lifestyle.
Acknowledge your responsibility to others to care for *your* health first.
Let those around you know your goals and support you every step of the way.

REAL DEAL Wellness Principles—THE BODY

REAL Action moves us.

Realize constant motion and action is the best way to keep body fat at bay.
Exercise daily—there are no days off from some form of physical activity.
Accept that your body changes only when you push out of your "comfort zone."
Learn new ways to physically challenge your body after reaching each goal.

REAL Nutrition feeds us.

Refuel your body to get through your workouts and daily physical activities.
Eat like your life depends on it, because it does.
Acknowledge what you're putting into your body and why—own your actions.
Let food do its job in your body. Stop attaching emotions and psychology to it.

REAL Maintenance renews us.

Refer to a physician for regular checkups to diagnose and treat conditions.
Enable your body to recuperate from exercise and get stronger with adequate rest.
Alleviate tightness and soreness by stretching muscles safely and routinely.
Learn how to perform self-exams* to aid in early detection of health conditions.

---

*(Consult your physician for the number, types and frequency of self-exams to perform based on your gender, age, lifestyle, family health history, etc.)

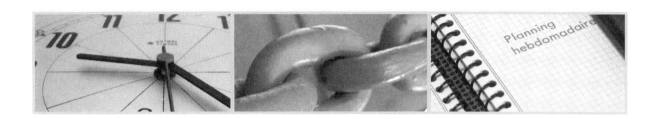

1. Prevention: A healthy lifestyle (eating right and exercise) is the ultimate form of prevention of health ailments.
2. Examination: Regular self-exams (men: testicular exams, women: breast exams) provide more frequent opportunities than yearly checkups to assess health status.
3. Detection: Annual physical checkups (more frequently for older people) help to detect health symptoms before they develop into full-blown conditions or diseases.

The successful treatment of many diseases depends on early detection. Give yourself the best odds by taking preventive measures like regular physical checkups, even if you supposedly "feel fine" and appear to be in good health. Looks can be deceiving. Medical science lets us see things we can't see. Hiding under our skin is a collection of tissues, cells, organs, bones and fluids doing what they do to keep us alive. Oftentimes, we can't see and, sometimes, we can't feel, when something is wrong. That's when we fall prey to "silent killers" like heart disease and high blood pressure. Save yourself the guesswork and see your doctor.

Address the body through nutrition and exercise. The following principles help enhance the feeding of your body and the strengthening of your body for a better overall quality of life.

REAL DEAL Wellness Principles—THE SPIRIT/SOUL

REAL Balance stabilizes us.
Release tension with healthy stress relievers to "center" you and keep you sane.
Engage in fulfilling hobbies and pastimes that contribute to your overall wellness.
Add discipline to your life—embrace what helps, eliminate what hinders.
Let self-control overrule unhealthy temptations that can throw you off balance.

REAL Passion fulfills us.
Relax/revive your spirit by enjoying passions that stimulate and fulfill you.
Express yourself through your passions and proudly leave a mark on the world.
Acquaint yourself with people that share your passions to gain perspective.
Love something or someone outside of yourself to "distribute" your passion.

REAL Spirituality enriches us.
Realize you're not alone in your quest to live a better life and honor the "source."
Embrace your uniqueness and let your spirit shine through your words and actions.
Analyze your contributions to the greater good of your community and the world.
Listen to the "voice" that speaks to you and encourages you through tough times.

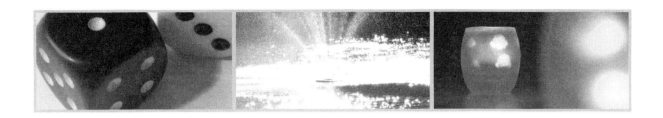

THE SPIRIT/SOUL

Stress management and spiritual nourishment complete your circle of health. Stress comes with the job of being alive. You can't eliminate aspects of your job description at work, and you cannot eliminate stress. You can only manage it. Stress is the body's physical reactions to change, and stress that goes unchecked can adversely affect your health. Mental and emotional stress can manifest themselves in physical complications and conditions, including ulcers, sleep disorders, weight gain or weight loss, weakened immune system and digestive problems. It can also be a contributing factor in conditions such as heart disease, high blood pressure, headaches and arthritis.

To reduce stress levels, try not to worry too much. Put things that concern you (family, work, money, health, etc.) into context and devise healthy ways to handle them, without resorting to dangerous means of coping (drug abuse, drinking, overeating, lashing out, etc.). Exercise is a great way to relieve tension and stress. Take out your frustrations on the weights and the Stairmaster. You'll feel better, stronger and more prepared to face your life's challenges.

Another way to keep your spirit balanced is to engage in fulfilling hobbies or passions (painting, dancing, knitting, listening or dancing to music, helping others, etc.). Some people honor the Source or Force of their lives and congregate with like-minded individuals with shared beliefs to uplift and nourish their souls. Whatever your path, find ways to keep your internal self healthy and motivated enough to take care of your external self. The result is a well-rounded you and a life that exemplifies wellness.

Address the spirit through enrichment and fulfillment. The following principles help enhance the feeding of your soul and the strengthening of your core for a positive outlook on life.

Applying the aforementioned general principles to the specifics of your life will fortify you and reaffirm your worthiness of the good things that come to you. Use *The REAL DEAL Personal Log* (page 91) to keep track of your lifestyle goals and personal progress toward wellness. Your coaches wish you good luck on your journey toward a life well lived. We'll be cheering for you and applauding the successes you are destined to achieve.

CONCLUSION
ONE LIFETIME = ONE JOURNEY

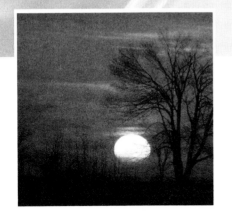

So, your tool kit for your lifestyle renovation is complete. The R.E.A.L. Concept teaches us that wellness is monitoring and balancing four basic elements of health: Rest (Recuperation), Exercise (Training), Appetite (Eating) and Lifestyle (Habits).

We utilize these tools to build our bodies and fix our lives. We learn what needs to be fixed and how to fix it by enacting *The REAL DEAL Four-Step Formula*: Wake up (Acknowledge), Get real (Accept), Take action (Act) and Get results (Achieve).

This is not the end. It is only the beginning. There is no timeframe or time limit for healthy living. Your goals should not stop with your upcoming cruise, reunion or wedding date. These big events are fine as kick-starters, but a first goal "to get started" should be followed by a second goal "to maintain." Once you get on the path to wellness, it becomes a lifestyle. Results start and stop when you do, so take just **ONE MINUTE** to get started.

Some people ask: "So, when do I know I'm totally fit, completely happy and thoroughly fulfilled with my life?" The answer: Like life, true health and fitness is a journey not a destination. As you take the journey, you may arrive at good health, but, to stay there, you must keep at it.

Fitness is forever; therefore, whether one is capable of reaching an "absolute or complete" version of it is uncertain. We all have work to do to reach our full potential in all areas of our lives. So don't seek so-called "perfection." It most likely will not surface. The best we can do is strive each day to be a little better, happier and healthier than we were the day before. Best wishes for a long and fruitful life. Stay fit!

REAL DEAL
TRAINING GUIDE REFERENCES

STRETCHING EXERCISES
Demonstrations & Descriptions

RESISTANCE TRAINING EXERCISES
Demonstrations & Descriptions

CARDIOVASCULAR/AEROBIC EXERCISES
Descriptions

REAL DEAL TRAINING LOG

REAL DEAL PERSONAL PROGRESS LOG

STRETCHING EXERCISES DEMONSTRATIONS & DESCRIPTIONS

Following are demonstrations and descriptions of the stretching exercises you can use to warm up your muscles before a workout or to wind down after exercise. When performing these exercises, follow the *Basic Stretching Exercise Tips* (page 6).

Lower Body Stretches

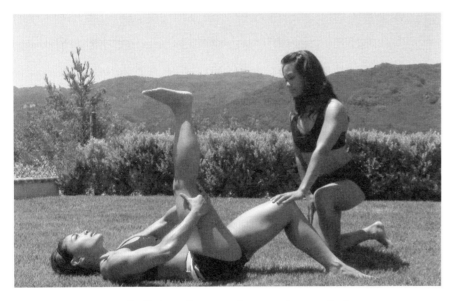

Hamstring Stretch: Lying down, raise one leg and clasp your hands behind your knee and pull the leg towards you until you feel a deep stretch in your hamstring (back of thigh) muscle. Hold the stretch. Relax and repeat with the opposite leg.

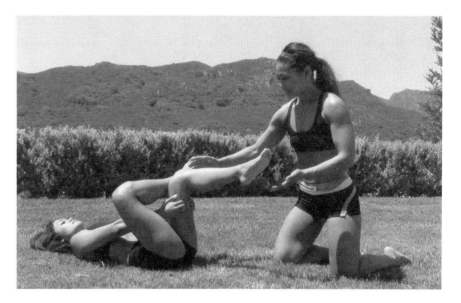

Glutes Stretch: Lying down, bend one knee at a 45-degree and rest the ankle of that leg on the opposite knee. Clasp your hands under the thigh of the leg that is still touching the floor. Pull your joined legs toward your chest until you feel a deep stretch in your glutes (buttocks). Hold the stretch. Relax, switch legs and repeat.

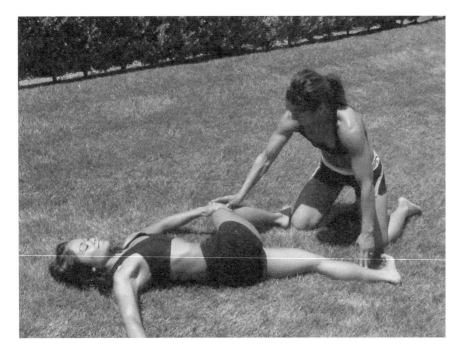 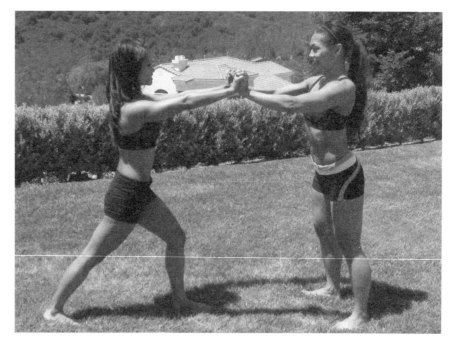

Hip & Lower-Back Stretch: Lying down, bend one knee at a 45-degree angle. With your hand, pull your bent knee (over the opposite thigh) toward the floor. until you feel a deep stretch in your lower back and the hip of the bent leg. Hold the stretch. Relax and repeat with the opposite leg.

Calf Stretch: Standing with your hands against a wall, extend your right leg backward and tuck your left foot behind the right ankle. Keeping your right leg straight and right heel pressed into the floor, lean forward until you feel a deep stretch in the calf of your right leg. Hold the stretch. Relax and repeat with the stretch with your left leg.

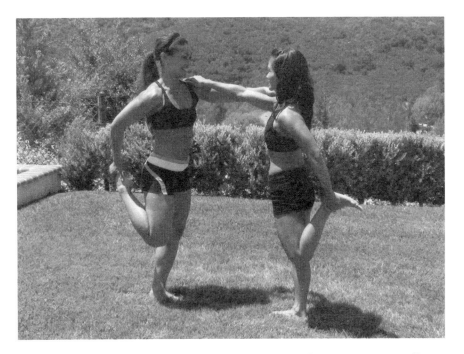
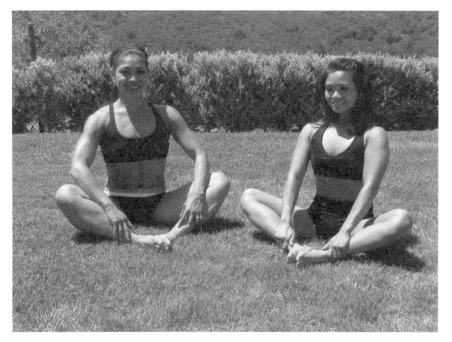

Quad/Thigh Stretch: Standing with one hand resting on a wall, bend one knee and grasp your foot with your free hand. Keeping your knees close to each other, pull your heel toward your buttocks until you feel a deep stretch in your quadriceps (thigh) muscle. Hold the stretch. Relax and repeat with the opposite leg.

"Butterfly Stretch" For Inner Thighs: Sitting on the floor with your knees bent outward and the soles of your feet pressed together, lean your upper body forward and place your bent elbows against the inner thighs. Use the weight of your upper body and elbows to push your knees toward the floor until you feel a deep stretch in your inner thighs. Hold the stretch. Relax and repeat.

UPPER BODY STRETCHES

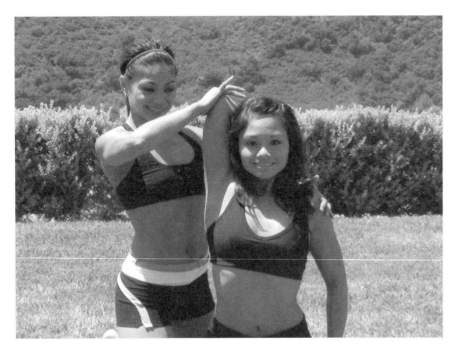

Triceps Stretch: Raise your right arm overhead, bend your elbow, and rest your hand behind your neck. Grasp your right elbow with your left hand and gently pull your elbow you feel a deep stretch in your right triceps. Hold the stretch. Relax and repeat with the stretch with your left arm.

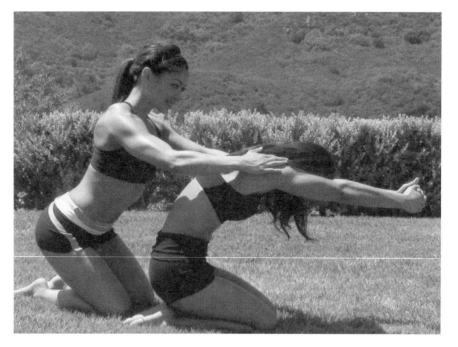

Upper-Back Stretch: Extend your arms at shoulder level and clasp your hands. Pushing your hands forward, spread your shoulder blades until your feel a deep stretch in your back. Hold the stretch. Relax and repeat.

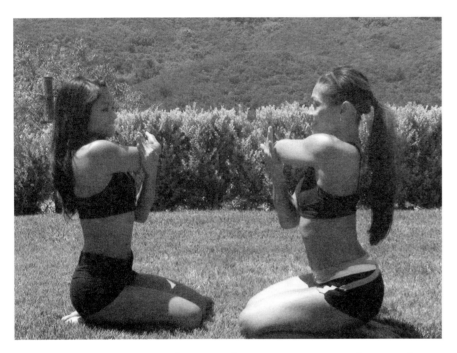 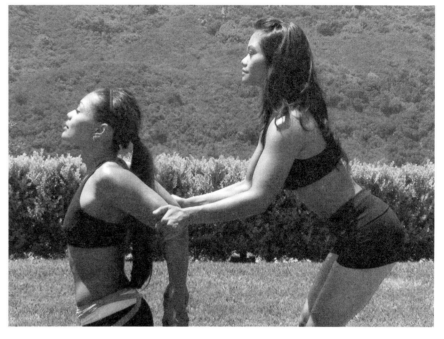

Shoulder Stretch: Extend your right arm across your chest and grasp your right elbow with your left hand. Gently pull your elbow toward your chest until you feel a deep stretch in your right shoulder. Hold the stretch. Relax and repeat with your left arm.

Pectoral (Chest) & Biceps Stretch: Place your hands on the sides of a doorway at shoulder height. Move your upper body forward until you feel a deep stretch in your biceps and across your pectoral (chest) muscles. Hold the stretch. This can also be performed one arm at a time, placing you right palm against a wall and rotating the rest of your body counter-clockwise (away from the wall). Then place your left palm on the wall while rotating your body clockwise.

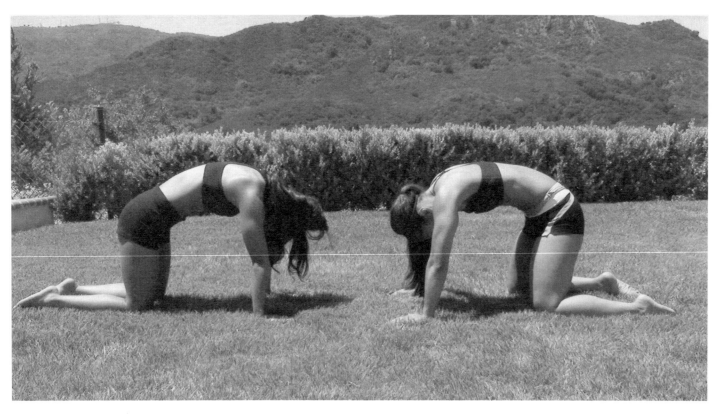

"Cat Stretch" For Back: Kneeling, place your hands on the floor and relax (sag) your back. Arch your spine (upward) like a cat until you feel a deep stretch in your back. Hold the stretch. Relax and repeat.

RESISTANCE TRAINING EXERCISES DEMONSTRATIONS & DESCRIPTIONS

Following are demonstrations and descriptions of the resistance training exercises you can use to design your workout program and strengthen the muscle groups. When performing these exercises, follow the *Basic Resistance Training Tips* (page 6).

BACK

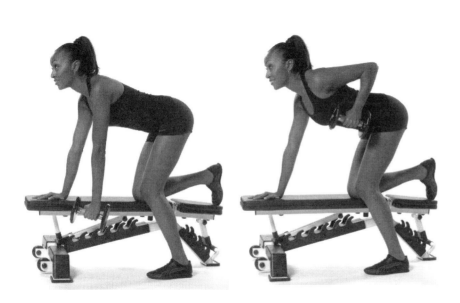

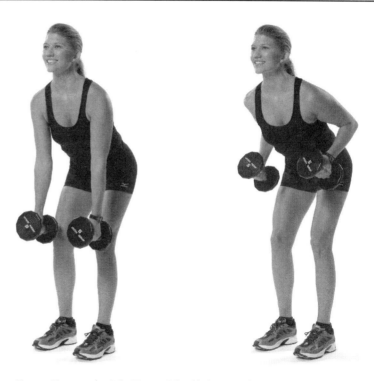

Single-Arm Rows: Leaning over a flat bench with your back flat, support yourself with one knee and one hand on the bench. Hold a dumbbell in your free hand. Squeezing your back, pull the dumbbell upward toward your ribcage until your bent elbow is above your back. Lower the dumbbell to the starting position then repeat. Complete a set on the opposite side, as well.

Bent-Over Rows (with Dumbbells): Bending over at the waist with your back nearly flat and knees slightly bent, hold a pair of dumbbells with your arms extended. Raising your elbows and squeezing your back muscles, pull the dumbbells upward toward your ribcage until your bent elbows are above your back. Lower the dumbbells to the starting position then repeat.

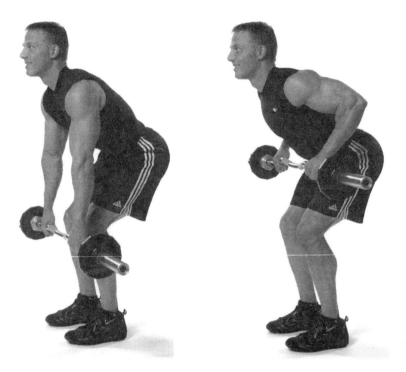

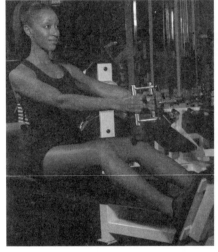 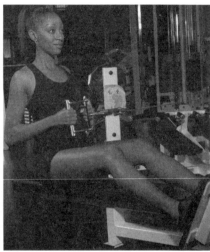

Bent-Over Rows (with Barbell): Bending over at the waist with your back nearly flat, knees slightly bent, hold a barbell with your arms extended Squeezing your back muscles, pull the barbell upward toward your ribcage until your bent elbows are above your back. Lower the barbell to the starting position then repeat.

Seated Rows (on Cable Row Machine): Sitting on a Cable Row machine with your back flat and feet planted on the footrests, hold the handle with your arms extended. Squeezing your back muscles, pull the handle toward your ribcage until your elbows are behind your back. Slowly release the handle forward to the starting position then repeat.

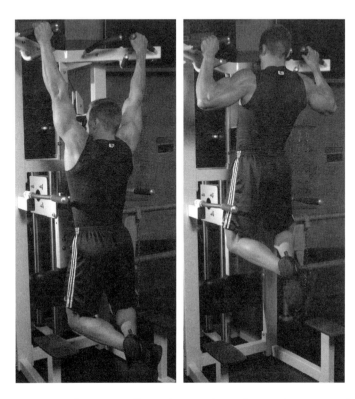

Pull-Ups: Hang from a pull-up bar with and a wide grip and arms extended. Squeezing your back muscles, pull your body upward until your chin reaches the bar. Lower your body to the starting position then repeat.

Pulldowns: (Not Pictured) Sitting upright at a pulldown machine, hold the overhead bar with a wide grip and your arms extended. Squeezing your back muscles, pull the bar down until it reaches your upper chest. Raise the bar to the starting position then repeat.

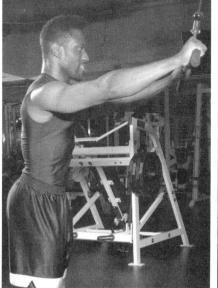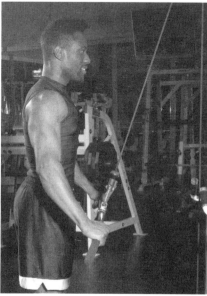

Straight-Arm Pulldowns:
Standing at a high-cable pulley with your back erect and arms extended, place flat palms on the bar at shoulder level. Squeezing your back muscles and keeping your arms straight, pull the bar down towards your thighs. Allow the bar to slowly rise to the starting position then repeat.

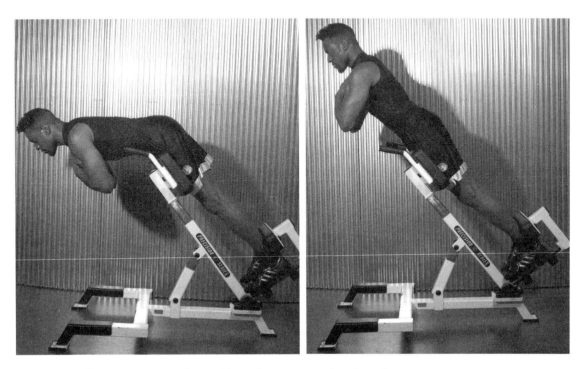

Lower-Back Hyperextensions: On a hyperextension bench, cross your arms over your chest and bend forward at the waist while keeping your back flat. Squeezing your lower back, raise your torso to the starting position then repeat. (Other options: Can also be performed with added resistance by holding weight against your chest.)

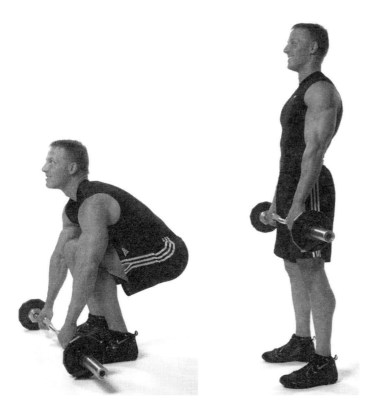

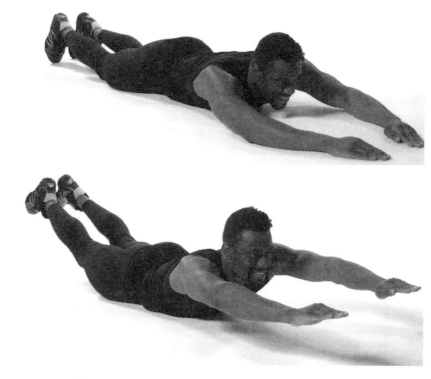

Deadlifts (for Lower Back): Starting in a crouched position with your back flat, hold a barbell with your arms extended toward the floor. Squeezing your lower back muscles, carefully straighten up tall. Slowly lower the barbell to the starting position then repeat.

Supermans (for Lower Back): Lying facedown, extend your arms overhead. Pressing your hips into the floor and squeezing your lower back muscles, raise your arms, chest and legs off the floor. Hold the position. Lower your limbs to the floor to the starting position then repeat.

CHEST

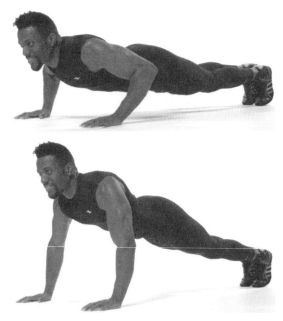

Pushups: Lying face-down, place your palms on the floor. Pushing with your chest muscles, extend your arms and lift your body to a plank position (balancing on your toes and palms). Bend your elbows to lower your body toward the floor then push your body back up and repeat. (Other options: Can also be performed with your knees remaining on the floor.)

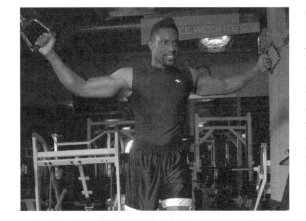

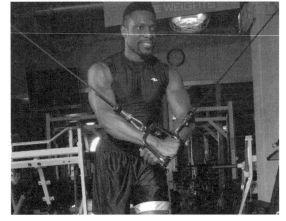

Cable Crossover: Standing between the weight stacks of a Cable Crossover machine, lean forward and balance yourself with one foot forward. In each hand, hold a handle attached to a high-cable pulley. Squeeze the chest muscles, pull the handles downward in a "hugging" motion. Allow the handles to return outward to the starting position then repeat.

Pec Deck: Sitting on a Pec Deck machine, back flat on the seatback, elbows bent at 90-degree angles, and forearms on the pads, squeeze your chest muscles and push the pads together. Allows the pads to return to the starting position then repeat.

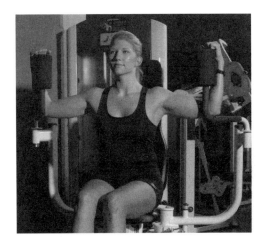

Dips (for Chest): (Not Pictured. See Dips for Triceps.) With your palms gripping parallel bars, hold your body up with extended arms. Bending your elbows, tilt your torso forward slightly and lower your body between the bars. Squeezing your chest muscles, extend your arms and push your body up to the starting position then repeat.

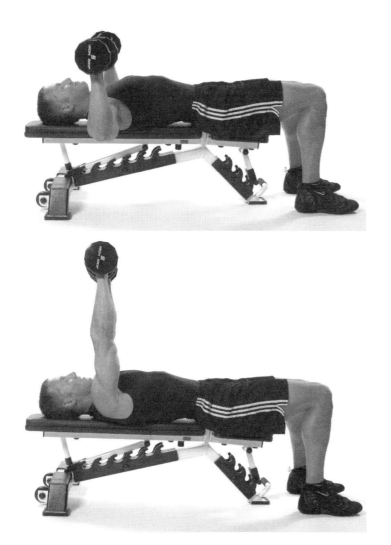

Flat Chest Presses: Lying on a flat bench, hold a pair of dumbbells, elbows bent at 90-degree angles. Squeezing your chest muscles, extend your arms and push the dumbbells up toward the ceiling. Lower the dumbbells to the starting position then repeat. (Other options: Can also be performed with a barbell.)

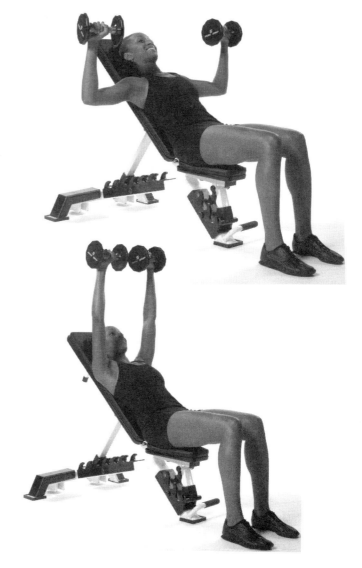

Incline Chest Presses: Reclining on an incline bench, hold a pair of dumbbells, elbows bent at 90-degree angles. Squeezing your upper chest, extend your arms and push the dumbbells up toward the ceiling. Lower the dumbbells to the starting position then repeat. (Other options: Can also be performed with a barbell.)

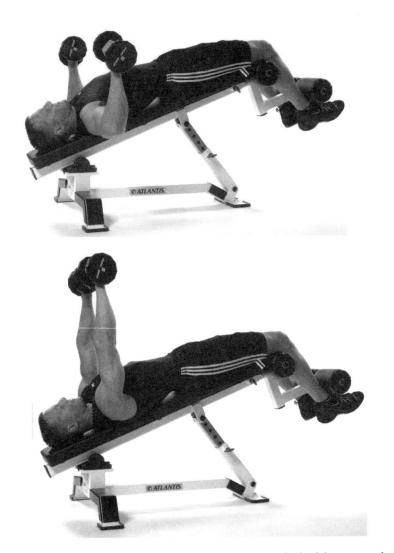
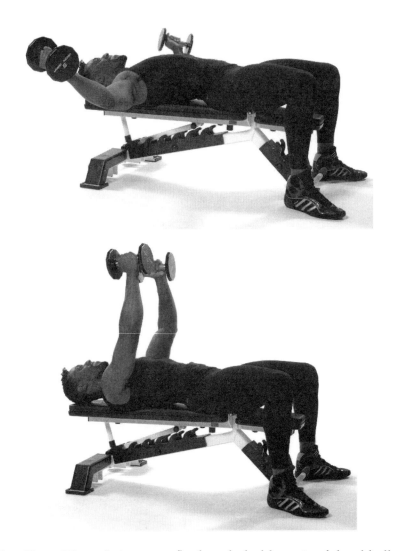

Decline Chest Presses: Lying on a decline bench, hold a pair of dumbbells, elbows bent at 90-degree angles. Squeezing your lower chest, extend your arms and push the dumbbells up toward the ceiling. Lower the dumbbells to the starting position then repeat. (Other options: Can also be performed with a barbell.)

Flat Chest Flyes: Lying on a flat bench, hold a pair of dumbbells above your chest, arms extended, palms facing each other. With slightly bent elbows, lower the dumbbells outward to your sides in a wide arching motion. Squeezing your chest muscles, raise the dumbbells to the starting position then repeat. (Other options: Can also be performed holding the handles of a Cable Crossover machine.)

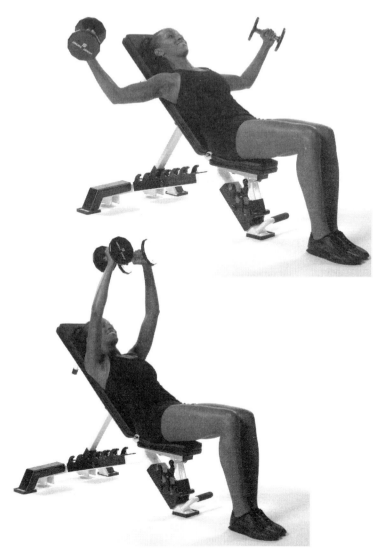
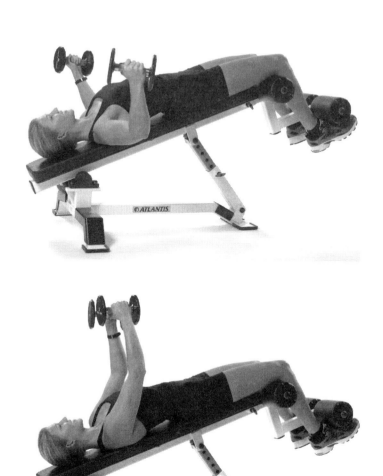

Incline Chest Flyes: Reclining on an incline bench, hold a pair of dumbbells above your upper chest, arms extended, palms facing each other. With slightly bent elbows, lower the dumbbells outward to your sides in a wide arching motion. Squeezing your chest muscles, raise the dumbbells to the starting position then repeat.

Decline Chest Flyes: Lying on a decline bench, hold a pair of dumbbells above your lower chest, arms extended, palms facing each other. With slightly bent elbows, lower the dumbbells outward to your sides in a wide arching motion. Squeezing your chest muscles, raise the dumbbells to the starting position then repeat.

SHOULDERS

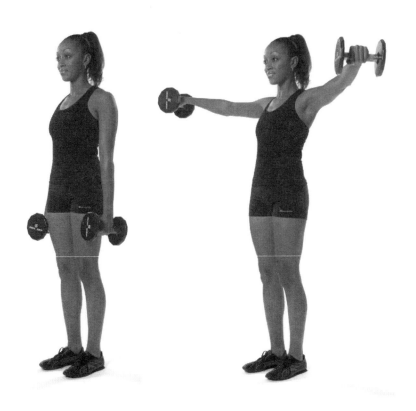 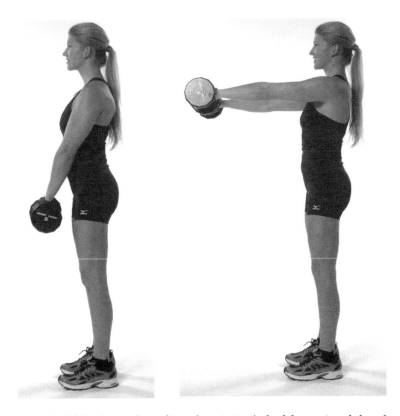

Lateral (Side) Deltoid Raises: Standing (or sitting), hold a pair of dumbbells at your sides. Squeezing your shoulder muscles, raise the dumbbells out to shoulder height. Lower the dumbbells to the starting position then repeat.

Front Deltoid Raises: Standing (or sitting), hold a pair of dumbbells at your sides. Squeezing your shoulder muscles, raise the dumbbells up to shoulder height. Lower the dumbbells to the starting position then repeat.

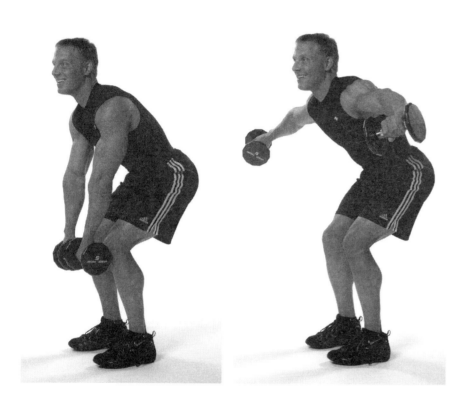
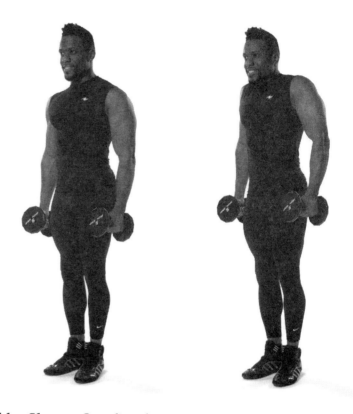

Rear Deltoid Raises: Standing (or sitting), bend forward at the waist. Hold a pair of dumbbells with your arms hanging straight down toward your feet. Squeezing your shoulder blades together, raise the dumbbells up toward the ceiling and parallel with your back. Lower the dumbbells to the starting position then repeat.

Shoulder Shrugs: Standing (or sitting on a bench), hold a pair of dumbbells at your sides. Squeezing the muscles that connect your neck and shoulders, raise the shoulders up toward your ears. Lower the dumbbells to the starting position then repeat.

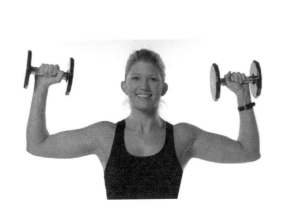 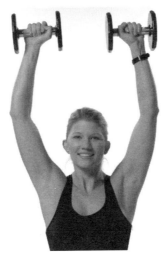

Shoulder Presses: Standing (or sitting), hold a pair of dumbbells at shoulder level, elbows at 90-degree angles. Squeezing your shoulder muscles, push the dumbbells up above your head until your arms are nearly straight. Lower the dumbbells to the starting position then repeat.

Upright Rows: Standing, hold a pair of dumbbells in front of you. Keeping the dumbbells close to your body, raise your elbows and pull the dumbbells up to your chin. Lower the dumbbells to the starting position then repeat.

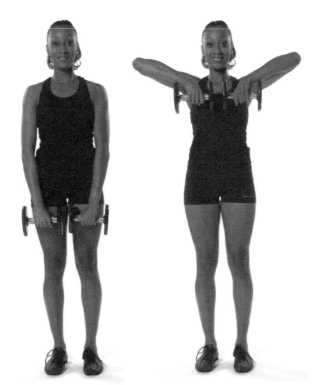 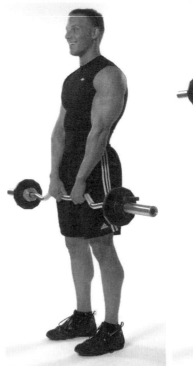 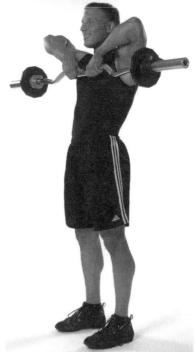

64   The One-Minute Workout

TRICEPS

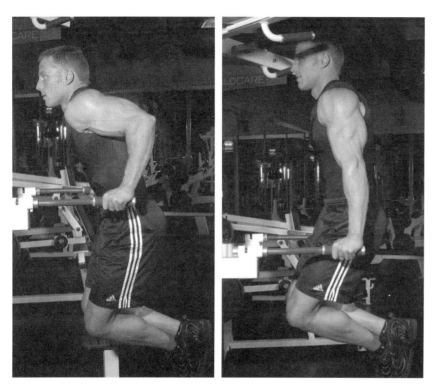

Dips (for Triceps): With your palms gripping parallel bars, hold your body up with extended arms. Bending your elbows, lower your body between the bars. Squeezing your chest muscles, extend your arms and push your body up to the starting position then repeat. (Other options: Can also be performed on a Dip Machine, particularly for those who cannot lift their own body weight.)

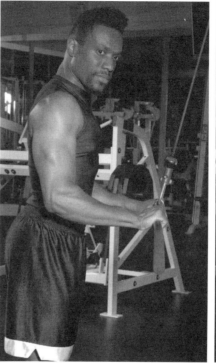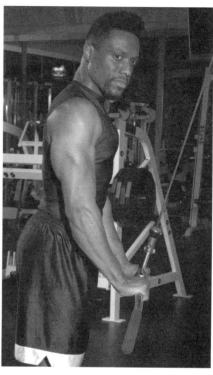

Triceps Pushdowns: Standing in front of a high-cable pulley, hold a bar attachment using an overhand grip with your arms close to your sides, elbows bent at 90-degree angles. Squeezing your triceps, extend your arms and push the bar down towards the floor. Allow the bar to rise to the starting position then repeat.

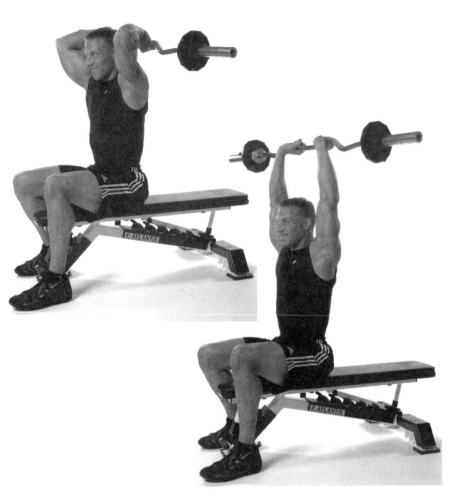 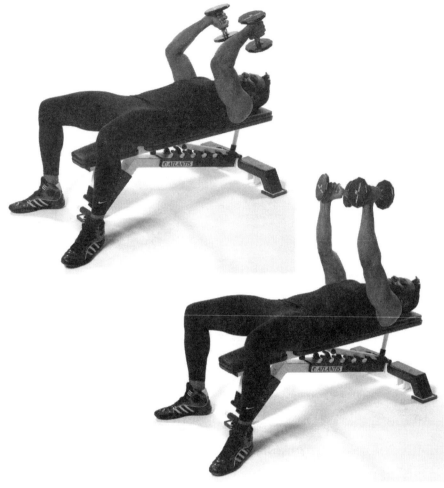

Overhead Triceps Extensions: Standing (or sitting), hold a barbell overheard. Bending your elbows, lower the barbell behind your head. Squeezing your triceps, extend your arms and raise the barbell up to the starting position, then repeat. (Other options: Can also be performed with one dumbbell or two dumbbells, or on an Overhead Triceps Extension machine.)

Lying Triceps Extensions (with Dumbbells): Lying down, hold a pair of dumbbells with your arms extended. Bending your elbows, lower the dumbbells back toward your ears. Squeezing your triceps, extend your arms and raise the dumbbells up to the starting position then repeat.

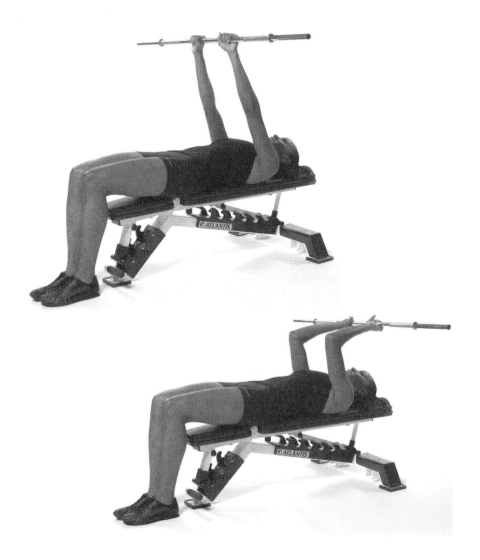

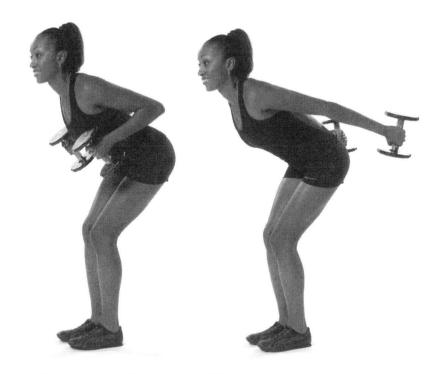

Bent-Over Triceps Extensions (Kickbacks): Bending over at the waist,, hold a pair of dumbbells with your arms against your sides, elbows bent at about 90-degree angles. Squeezing your triceps, raise the dumbbells until your arms are parallel with the floor. Bending your elbows, lower the dumbbells to the starting position then repeat.

Lying Triceps Extensions (with Barbell): Lying down, hold a barbell with your arms extended. Bending your elbows, lower the barbell back toward your forehead. Squeezing your triceps, extend your arms and raise the barbell up to the starting position then repeat.

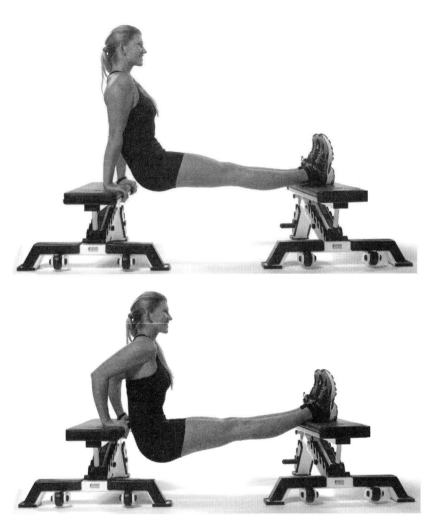

Bench Dips: Suspend your body between two benches, supporting yourself with your palms on one bench and your feet on the other bench. Bending your elbows, lower your body. Squeezing your triceps, extend your arms and push your body up to the starting position then repeat. (Other options: Can also be performed with your hands on one bench and your feet on the floor.)

BICEPS

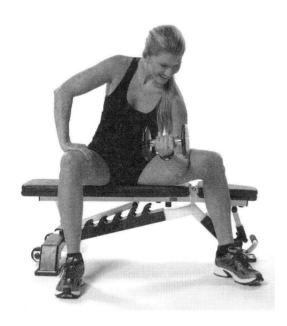
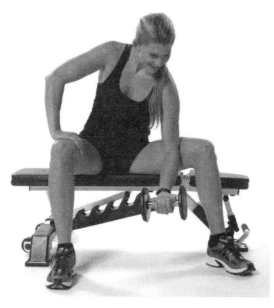

Concentration Curls: Sitting with your torso leaning forward, hold a dumbbell in one hand and place your elbow against your inner thigh. Rest your free hand on your other knee for support. Flexing your biceps, curl the dumbbell upward. Lower the dumbbell to the starting position then repeat. Complete a set with the opposite arm.

Incline Dumbbell Curls: Reclining on an incline bench, hold a pair of dumbbells with your arms dangling at your sides. Flexing your biceps, curl the dumbbells upward, while keeping your elbows stationary. Lower the dumbbells to the starting position then repeat.

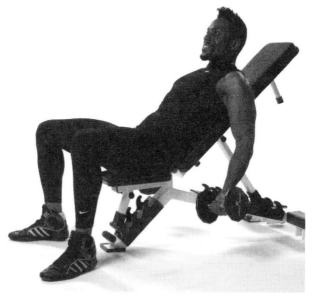
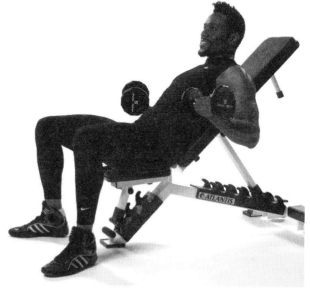

Training Guide References

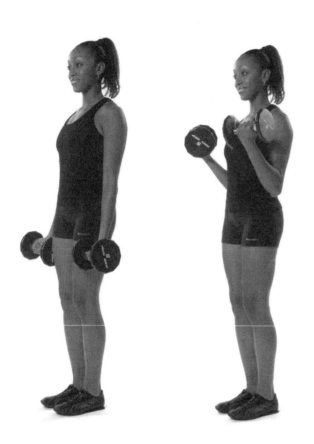

Dumbbell Curls: Standing (or sitting), hold a pair of dumbbells at your sides. Flexing your biceps, curl the dumbbells upwards, while keeping your elbows close to your sides. Lower the dumbbells to the starting position then repeat.

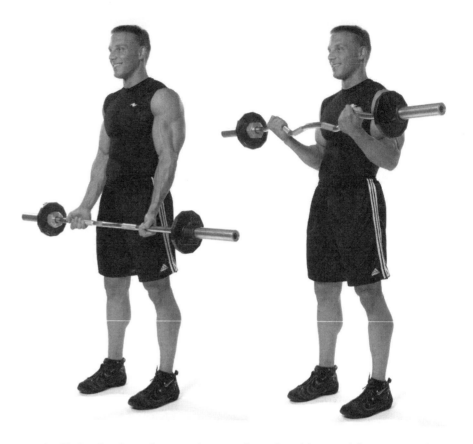

Barbell Curls: Standing with your feet shoulder-width apart and arms extended, hold a barbell in front of using an underhand grip. Contracting your biceps while keeping your elbows tight and stationary, curl the barbell up to shoulder level, without swinging or rocking your torso. Lower the barbell to the starting position, then repeat.

Preacher Curls: (Not Pictured) Sitting at a preacher curl bench, hold a barbell with an underhand grip and your elbows against the pad. Flexing your biceps, curl the barbell upward to your chin. Slowly lower the barbell to the starting position then repeat.

QUADRICEPS

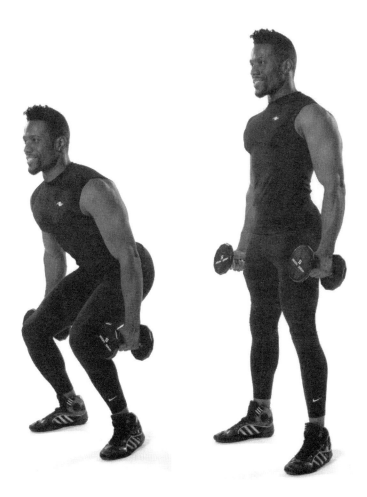 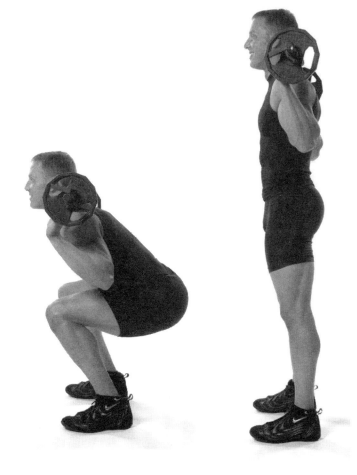

Squats (Traditional, with Dumbbells): Standing with your feet apart, hold a pair of dumbbells at your sides. Keeping your head and chest up, bend your knees and squat to a sitting positing. Squeezing your glutes and thigh muscles, extend your legs until you are standing in the starting position then repeat.

Squats (Traditional, with Barbell): Standing with your feet apart, rest a barbell across your shoulders. Keeping your head and chest up, bend your knees and squat to a sitting positing. Squeezing your glutes and thigh muscles, extend your legs until you are standing in the starting position then repeat.

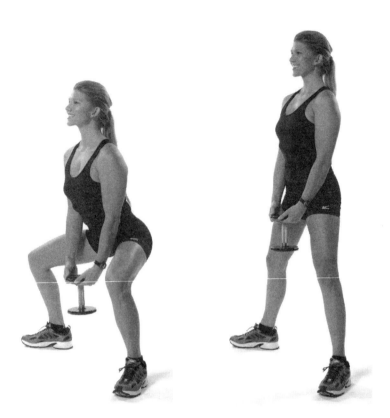
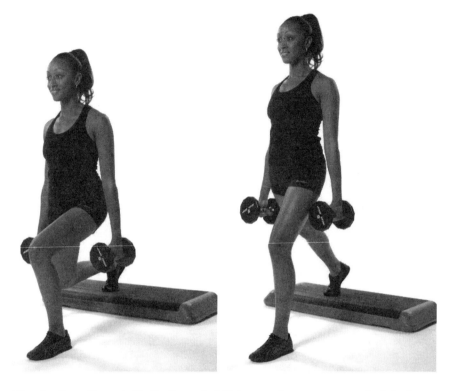

Sumo Squats: Standing in a wide stance, hold a dumbbell in front of you. Lowering the dumbbell as you squat, bend your knees, drop your hips and buttocks backward (while keeping your head and chest up), to a sitting position. Squeezing your glutes and thigh muscles, extend your legs until you are standing in the starting position then repeat.

Single-Leg Squat (Split Squat): With one foot on a step behind you and your other foot flat on the floor in front of you, hold a pair of dumbbells at your sides. Bending your front knee, squat down until your thigh is parallel with the floor. Squeezing your glutes and thigh muscles, extend your front leg until you are standing in the starting position then repeat. Switch legs and complete another set. (Other options: Can also be performed with both feet on the floor.)

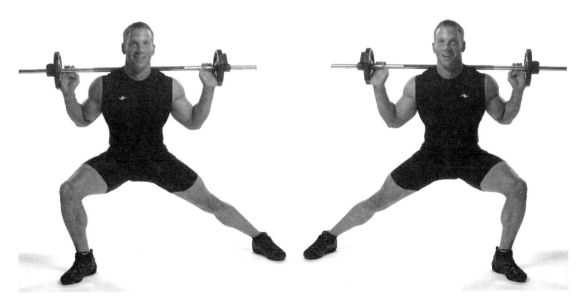

Wide-Stance Side-to-Side Squats: Standing in wide stance, rest a barbell across your shoulders. Bending your left knee, squat down to your left side until you feel a deep stretch in your right inner thigh. Squeezing your glutes and left thigh muscles, extend your left leg. Next, squat to your right side. Tightening your glutes and right thigh muscles, extend your right leg. Repeat, alternating.

Lunges (Stationary): Standing with your feet together, hold a pair of dumbbells at your sides. Lunging one foot forward in a long stride, bend the knee until your thigh is parallel with the floor (while bending the knee of the rear leg toward the floor). Squeezing your thigh muscles and pushing up with your heel, extend your front leg and until you are standing in the starting position then repeat. Complete a set with the opposite leg. (Other options: Can also be performed walking in a forward path with each lunge.)

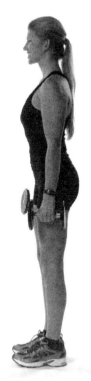
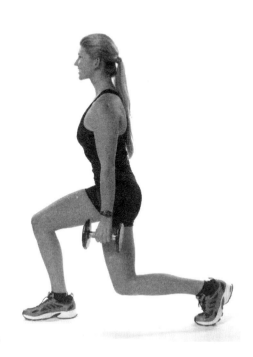

Training Guide References

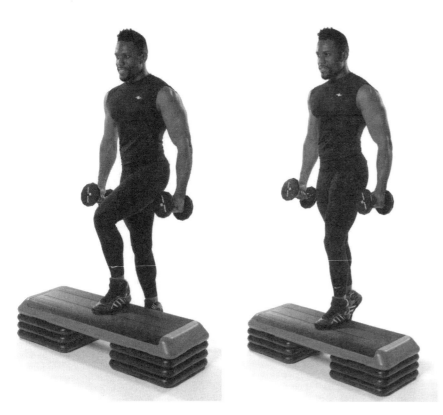

Step-Ups: Standing in front of a high step/bench, hold a pair of dumbbells. Place one foot on the step/bench. Squeezing your glutes and thigh muscles, step up onto the step/bench. Step backward onto the floor one foot at a time until you are standing in the starting position, then repeat, leading with the opposite foot.

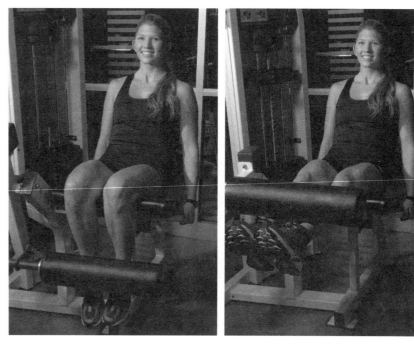

Leg Extensions: Sitting on a Leg Extension machine, keep your back erect and pressed against the seatback and place your feet under the footpad. Squeezing your thigh muscles, extend your legs and raise the footpad. Bending your knees, lower the footpad to the starting position then repeat.

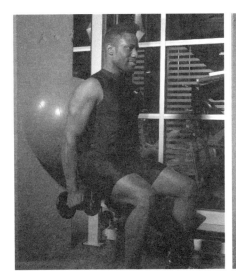
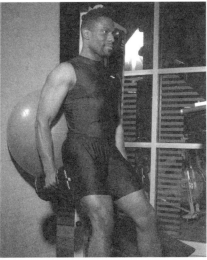
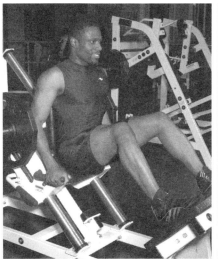
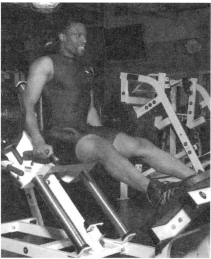

Exercise Ball Squats: Standing with your feet apart and your lower back on an exercise ball resting against a wall, hold a pair of dumbbells. Bend your knees, letting the ball roll up your spine as you squat down to a sitting position. Squeezing your glutes and thigh muscles, extend your legs as the ball rolls back down your spine until you are standing in the starting position then repeat.

Hack Squats: Reclining on a Hack Squat machine with your shoulders against the pads of the sled (or, on certain machines, sitting on the sled's seat), place your feet on the platform. Bending your knees, squat down to a sitting position. Squeezing your glutes and thigh muscles, extend your legs and raise the sled until you are standing in the starting position then repeat.

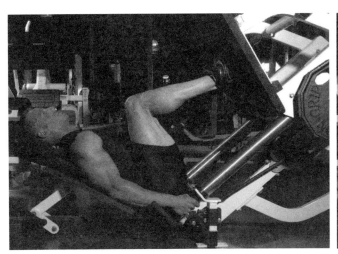
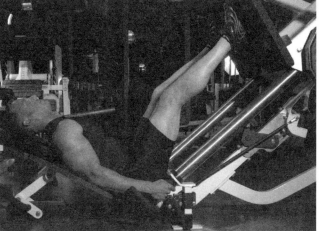

Leg Presses: Lying on a decline Leg Press machine (or sitting on a horizontal Leg Press machine), place your feet on the platform. Bending your knees, lower the platform (or the seat, on some horizontal machines) to a comfortable level. Squeezing your glutes and thigh muscles, push with your heels and extend your legs to raise the platform (or seat) to the starting position then repeat.

Training Guide References **75**

BUTTOCKS (GLUTES)

Glute Kickbacks (Donkey Kicks): Kneeling on the floor, support your upper body with your hands (or elbows) on the floor. Raise one leg behind you with your knee bent and your foot flexed. Squeezing your glutes, extend your raised leg, kicking it upward toward the ceiling. Lower your leg to the starting position then repeat. Complete a set with the opposite leg.

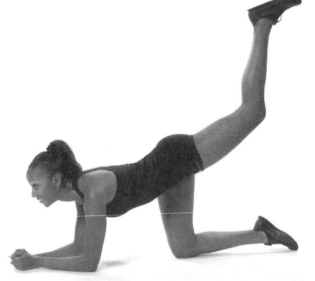

Hip Thrusts (Bridges): Lying down, bend your knees and keep your feet flat on the floor. Squeezing your glutes, thrust your hips up until you form a slanted "bridge" with your body (knees up, shoulders down). Dropping your hips, lower your body to the starting position then repeat.

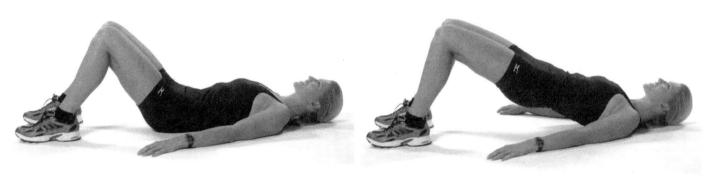

Glute Master: (Not Pictured) Kneeling on a Glute Master machine, support your upper body with your hands (or elbows) on the arm pads. Raise one leg behind you with your knee bent and your foot flexed on the footrest. Squeezing your glutes, extend your raised leg, kicking it upward toward the ceiling. Lower your leg to the starting position then repeat. Complete a set with the opposite leg.

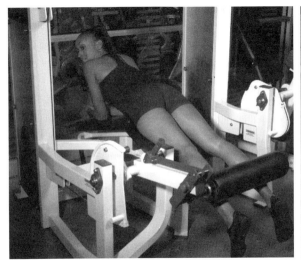
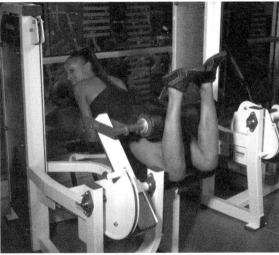
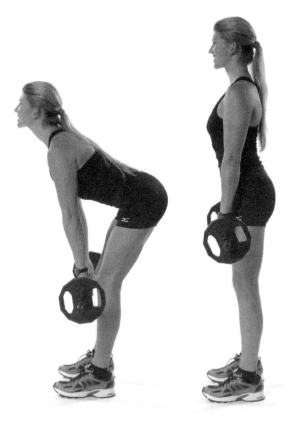

Lying Leg Curls: Lying facedown on a Leg Curl machine, place your feet under the footpad. Squeezing your hamstrings, bend your knees and curl the footpad up toward your glutes. Lower the footpad to the starting position then repeat. (Other options: Can also be performed on a Seated Leg Curl machine or a Standing Leg Curl machine.)

Stiff-Legged Deadlifts (for Hamstrings): Bending over at the waist with your back flat and knees locked, hold a barbell with your arms extended toward the floor. Squeezing your hamstring muscles, carefully straighten up tall. Bending over, slowly lower the barbell to the starting position then repeat. (Other options: Can also be performed with dumbbells.)

INNER/OUTER THIGH

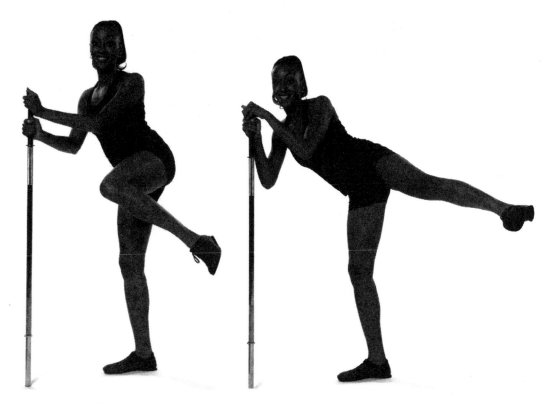

Karate Kicks (for Hips & Outer Thighs): Leaning sideways against a stationary object, balance yourself on one leg and raise the other leg until it is parallel with the floor. Bend the knee of the raised leg inward toward your body. Foot flexed, kick your leg out to the starting position then repeat. Complete a set with the opposite leg.

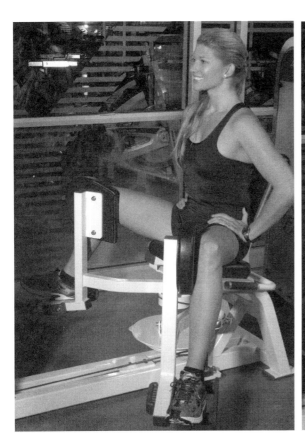 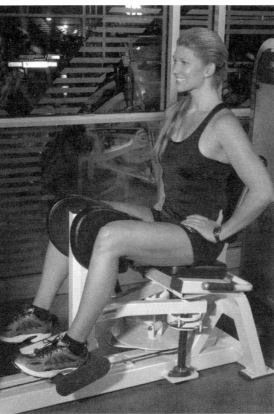

Adductor: Sitting on an Adductor machine, place your knees on the kneepads. Squeezing your inner thighs, use your knees to push the kneepads inward until they meet in the center. Parting your thighs, allow the kneepads to move outward to the starting position then repeat.

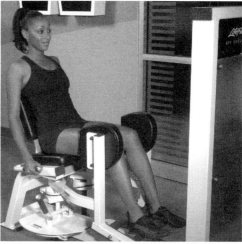
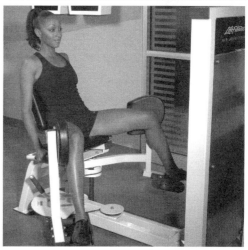

Abductor: Sitting on an Abductor machine, place your knees on the kneepads. Tightening your outer thighs, use your knees to push the kneepads outward and squeeze your glutes. Closing your thighs, allow the kneepads to move inward together to the starting position then repeat.

Training Guide References **79**

CALVES

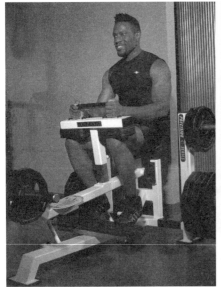 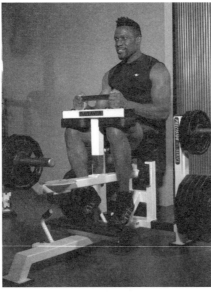

Seated Calf Raises: Sitting on a Seated Calf Raise machine, tuck your legs under the kneepads and place the balls of your feet on the footrest. Stretching your calf muscles, lower your heels. Flex your feet, rise up high on your toes, and squeeze your calves. Lower your heels to the starting position then repeat.

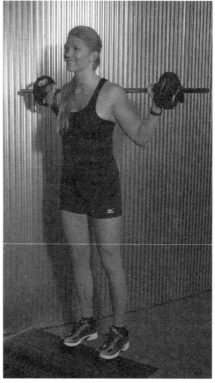 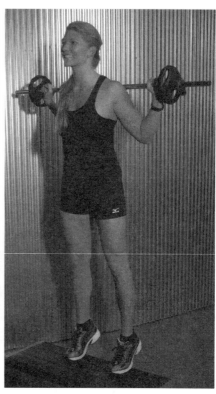

Standing Calf Raises: Standing on a Standing Calf Raise machine, position your shoulders under the shoulder pads and place the balls of your feet on the footrest. Stretching your calf muscles, lower your heels. Flex your feet, rise up high on your toes and flex your calves. Lower your heels to the starting position then repeat. (Other options: Can also be performed holding a barbell or dumbbells while standing on a step.)

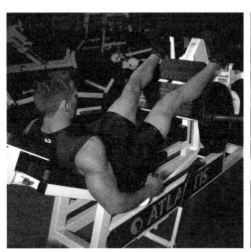 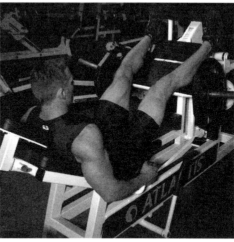

Calf Presses on Leg Press Machine: Lying on an incline Leg Press machine or sitting on a horizontal Leg Press machine, place the balls of your feet on the platform. Flexing your feet and pushing with your toes to raise the platform (or seat), squeeze your calves. Lower your heels to the starting position then repeat.

ABS/CORE

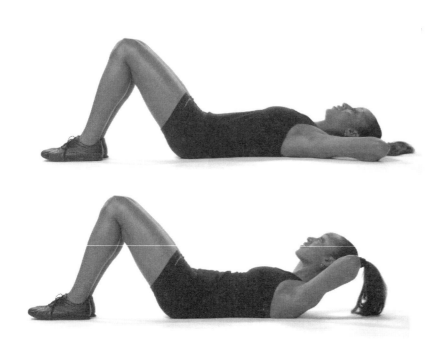

Traditional Crunches: Lying down, bend your knees and place your feet flat on the floor. With your hands behind your ears, press your lower back into the floor as you lift your chest, and squeeze your abdominal muscles. Lower your upper body to the starting position then repeat. (Other options: Can also be performed with added resistance by holding weight behind your head or on your chest.)

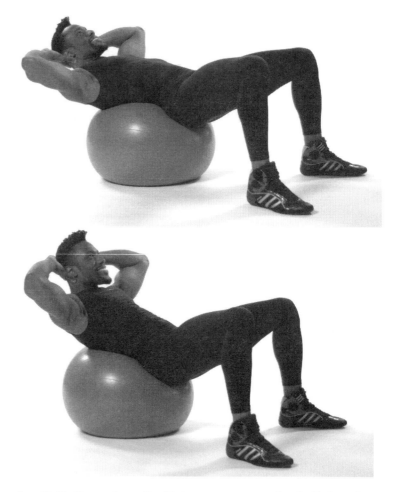

Exercise Ball Crunches: Reclining on an exercise ball, bend your knees and place your feet flat on floor. With your hands behind your ears, lift your chest and squeeze your abdominal muscles. Lower your upper body to the starting position then repeat. (Other options: Can also be performed with added resistance by holding weight behind your head or on your chest.)

Scissor Kicks: Lying down, keep your extended legs lifted a few inches off the floor. Squeezing your abdominal muscles, kick your feet up and down, moving your legs in a rapid "scissor-like" motion. Repeat for several repetitions.

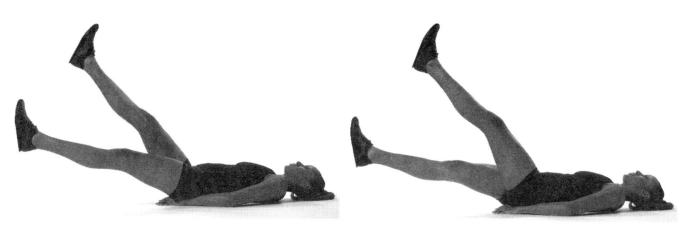

Reverse (Low-Ab) Crunches: Lying down, bend your knees and keep your feet raised off the floor. Extend your arms to your sides (or tuck your hands under glutes). Squeezing your lower abdominal muscles and lifting your hips, roll your pelvis forward until your knees nearly touch your chest. Lower your legs to the starting position then repeat.

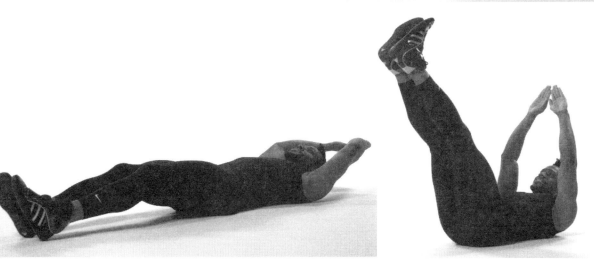

Jackknife Sit-Ups: Lying down with your extended legs together, raise your arms overhead. Squeezing your abdominal muscles, raise your straight arms and straight legs toward each other in a "jackknife" motion. Lower your arms and legs to the starting position then repeat.

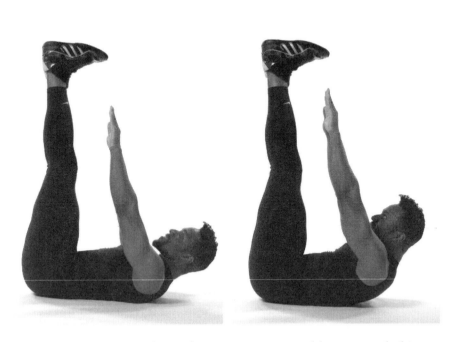

Toe Touchers: Lying down, keep your arms and legs extended in a vertical position. Squeeze your abdominal muscles as you lift your torso to reach for your toes. Lower your upper body to the starting position then repeat.

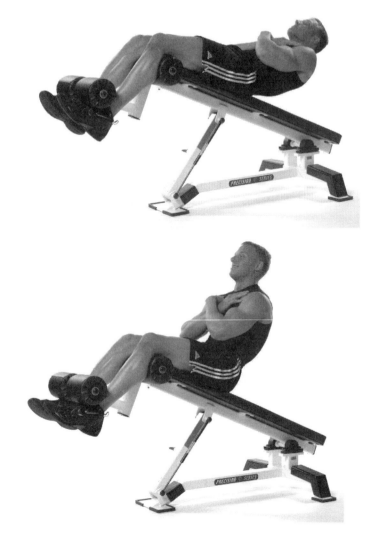

Decline Bench Crunches: Reclining on a decline bench, leave your upper body raised off the bench to keep constant tension on your abdominal muscles. With your hands behind your ears, squeeze your abs and lift your upper body. Recline to the starting position then repeat.

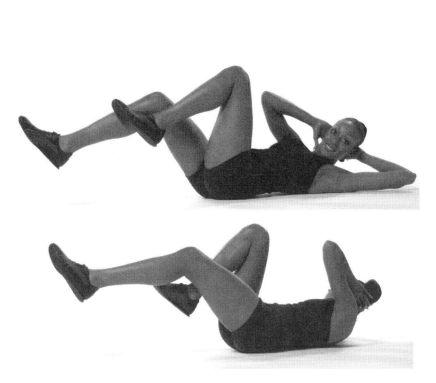

Air Bicycle: Lying down, raise your feet up in the air with your knees bent at 90-degree angles and place your hands behind your ears. Swiftly extend and bend your legs in a cyclical motion as if you are riding a bicycle. Squeezing your abdominal muscles, lift your torso slightly and twist it from side to side as you touch each elbow to the opposite knee in a constant, alternating fashion.

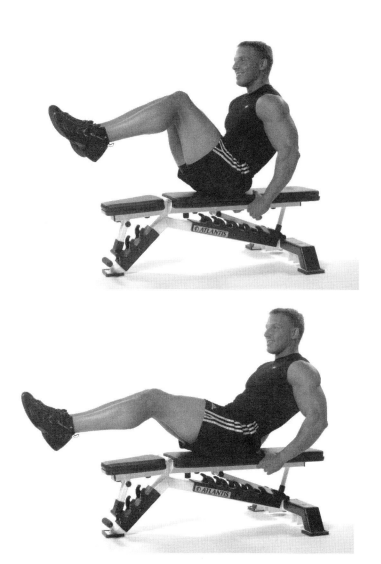

Seated Flat-Bench Leg Pull-Ins: Sitting on the end of a flat bench, lift your extended legs parallel to the floor. Lean back to keep constant tension on your abdominal muscles. Hold on to the sides of the bench for light support. Squeezing your lower abdominal muscles, pull your knees inward toward your chest. Extend your legs to the starting position then repeat.

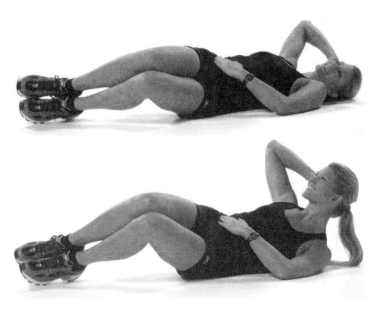

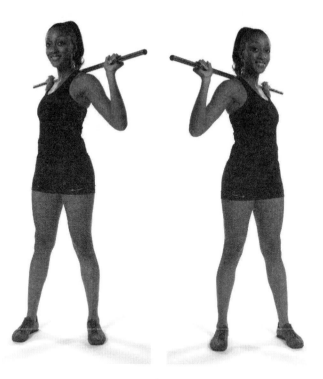

Oblique Twists: Standing with a wide stance, hold a bar across your shoulders. Keep your head up, and your hips stationary. Twisting at your waist, rotate your torso (and the bar) from right to the left. Repeat for several repetitions.

Oblique Crunches: Lying on your right side with your knees bent, place your left hand behind your left ear. Squeezing your obliques, lift your torso up toward the ceiling. Lower your upper body to the starting position then repeat. Complete a set on the opposite side.

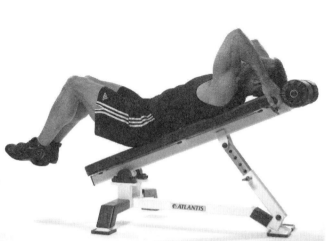
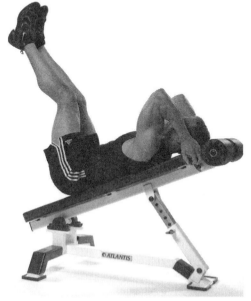

Decline Reverse Crunches: Lying on a decline bench, hold on to the top of the bench and extend your legs parallel to the floor. Squeezing your lower abdominal muscles, raise your legs to a vertical position. Lower your legs to the starting position then repeat. (Other options: Can also be performed with bent knees.)

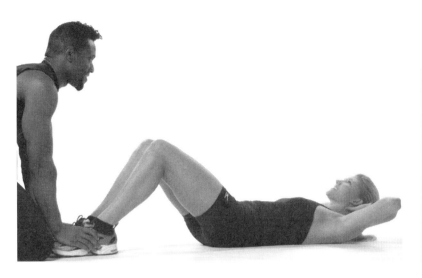 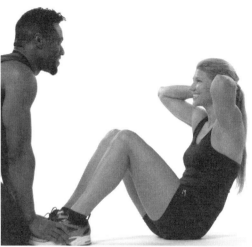

Sit-Ups: Lying down, bend your knees and tuck your feet under a stationary object (or have them held down by a partner). With your hands behind your ears (or with your arms crossed over your chest), bend at the waist and squeeze your abdominal muscles as you lift your torso to sit up vertically. Lower your torso to the starting position then repeat.

Flat-Bench Lying Leg Raises: Lying on a flat bench, tuck your hands under glutes and extend your legs parallel to the floor. Squeezing your lower abdominal muscles, lift your legs to a vertical position. Lower your legs to the starting position then repeat. (Other options: Can also be performed with bent knees.)

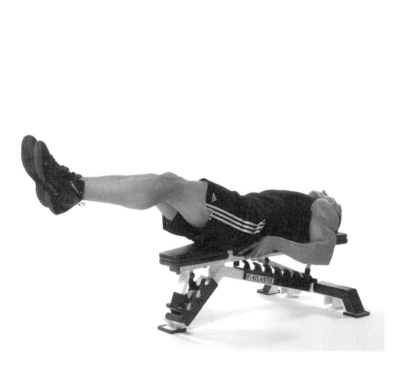 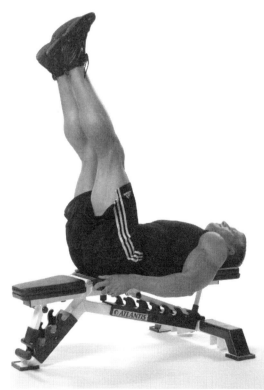

Training Guide References **87**

CARDIOVASCULAR/AEROBIC EXERCISES DESCRIPTIONS

Following is a list of cardiovascular/aerobic exercises you can use to design your workout program, increase fat-burning potential and improve your heart and lung health. When performing these exercises, follow the *Basic Cardiovascular/Aerobic Training Tips* (page 7).

CARDIO EXERCISES FOR ONE-MINUTE WORKOUT PROGRAMS

Squat Thrusts
Jump in the air. As you land on your feet, bend your knees and squat. From the squat position place your hands on the floor and thrust your legs behind you until you are in a horizontal, push-up position. In continuous motion, pull your knees in, plant your feet, lift your hands from the floor and rise, jumping in the air again. Repeat.

Step-Ups
Step up and down on a bench or step, alternating your feet each time.

Jumping Squats
Jump in the air. As you land on your feet, bend your knees and squat. As you rise, leap in the air. Repeat

Jumping Jacks
Continuously jumping, swing your arms out and above your head, while you land with your legs apart and your feet in a wide stance. Then jump again, dropping your arms down to your sides and landing with your legs and feet together. Repeat.

Sprinting
Take short, explosive runs from a starting location to an end location and back again.

Jumping Rope
Continuously jumping, hold the handles of a jump rope and circulate the rope around your body, over your head and under your feet with brisk revolutions.

Running Stairs
Jog up and down a staircase at a brisk pace.

Jumping Lunges
Jump in the air then softly land in a lunge position with your right foot planted on the floor and your left knee pointing toward the floor. Rising, jump in the air again and land in a lunge position with your left foot planted on the floor and your right knee pointing toward the floor. Alternate with each jump.

Running/Jogging
Run or jog from a starting location to an end location and back again. Or jog "in place" (in a stationary spot, kicking your knees high).

Step Footwork
Use a Step Aerobics step to perform a mix of step-ups, jogging up and down the step, and lunges off the side of the step.

Side-to-Side Shuffling
With knees slightly bent and your body in a low, semi-squat position, shuffle your feet sideways for a count of five, carrying your body to the left. Then shuffle your feet sideways for a five counts back to the right.

Treadmill
Jog, run or sprint on the treadmill.

Stationary Bike
Ride the stationary bike for "a sprint," i.e., using quick revolutions of your feet on the pedals.

GENERAL CARDIO EXERCISES

Cycling	StairMaster	Recumbent Bike
Kickboxing	Calisthenics	SkiingPlyometrics\
Rowing	Sprinting	Brisk Walking
Jumping Rope	Sport-Specific Drills	Running Stairs
Swimming	Racquetball	Running/Jogging
Step Footwork	Tennis	Elliptical Trainer
Treadmill	Yoga	Basketball
Martial Arts	Boxing	Pilates
Soccer	Hiking	

REAL DEAL TRAINING LOG

Track your Cardio, Resistance Training and Total Body Workouts.

These are basic principles to keep in mind as you plan your training program:

Basic Real Deal Training Principles

Repair/rejuvenate your body with rest.
Elevate your metabolic rate with cardio exercise.
Activate your muscles with resistance training.
Loosen/lengthen your body with stretching exercises.

Date: _____/_____/_____

Day: M T W Th F Sat Sun *(circle one)*   Time:_____

Goals

For the day:_____

Long-term:_____

Cardio Training

Exercise(s):_____

Intensity Level:_____

Total Time (Duration):_____

Total Body Training

No. of Exercises per Muscle Group(s):_____

No. and Duration of Aerobic Intervals:_____

Total Time (Duration):_____

Resistance Training

Target Muscle Group(s):_____

Exercise   Weight   Sets   Reps

_____

_____

_____

_____

_____

_____

_____

Notes

Did you:
Warm up?____ Cool down?____ Stretch?____ *(check reminder)*

Rate your Intensity Level: circle: *(low)* 1 2 3 4 5 *(high)*

Satisfied with your workout?
Yes?____ No?____ Somewhat?____ *(check one)*

Miscellaneous Notes:_____

_____

_____

_____

(Make photocopies of this page, collect them for your records and refer to them as a motivational tool.)

REAL DEAL PERSONAL PROGRESS LOG

Track your goals and personal progress periodically.

These are basic principles to keep in mind as you plan your lifestyle program:

Basic Real Deal Lifestyle Principles

Reduce stress.
Enjoy a hobby/passion.
Allocate time for yourself.
Listen to your soul and/or spirituality source.

Date: _____/_____/_____

Day: M T W Th F Sat Sun *(circle one)*   Time:_____

Fitness Goal 1

I will:_____

By (Month/Day/Year):_____ How?_____

Fitness Goal 2

I will:_____

By (Month/Day/Year):_____ How?_____

Personal Goal 1

I will:_____

By (Month/Day/Year):_____ How?_____

Personal Goal 2

I will:_____

By (Month/Day/Year):_____ How?_____

Notes

Current Fitness Level:
Novice____   Intermediate____   Advance____   *(check one)*

Rate Personal Satisfaction Level: *(low)* 1 2 3 4 5 *(high)*

Rate Current Stress Level: *(low)* 1 2 3 4 5 *(high)*

Significant Dates/Events/Commitments:_____
_____
_____

Personal Days & "Me Time" Appointments:_____
_____
_____

Miscellaneous Notes:_____
_____
_____
_____

(Make photocopies of this page, collect them for your records and refer to them as a motivational tool.)

REAL DEAL
EATING GUIDE REFERENCES

RULE 1 • MIX IT UP! (VARIETY)
More or Less List
Nutrition Facts Labels

RULE 2 • GET CARB SMART! (CARBS)
Glycemic Index

RULE 3 • AVOID BAD FAT! (FATS)
LDL vs. HDL Cholesterol

RULE 4 • BURN YOUR FOOD! (CALORIES)
5 REAL Keys to Weight Management

REAL DEAL EATING LOG

RULE 1 • Mix It Up!

MORE OR LESS LIST

So, how do you "mix it up?" Here is a handy *More or Less List* to help you apply the first nutrition Rule and add variety to your eating program.

Eat More	Eat Less
Fruits & Vegetables	
• Fresh, frozen, canned, dried	• Prepared in butter or sauces
Breads & Cereals	
• Whole-grain breads and cereals • Rice and pasta • Low-fat baked products • Baked goods containing minimal unsaturated oils	• Breads with eggs as a major ingredient • Egg noodles • Commercially baked products: pies, cakes • doughnuts, pastries, croissants, etc.
Fats & Oils	
• Unsaturated vegetable oils: sunflower corn, sesame, soybean, olive • Regular or diet margarine • Low-fat mayonnaise & salad dressings of recommended oils • Baking cocoa • Seeds & nuts	• Butter, coconut oil, palm oil, lard & bacon fat canola, safflower, • Dressings made with egg yolk • Chocolate • Coconut
Fish, Poultry, Meat & Vegetable Protein	
• Fish, poultry without skin, lean meats & vegetable proteins, such as beans, peas	• Fatty cuts of meat, cold cuts, sausage, hot dogs, bacon, sardines, roe & beans prepared & tofu with lard
Dairy Products	
• Skim or 1% milk, low-fat buttermilk & cottage cheese • Nonfat or low-fat yogurt or (no more than 2-4 grams of fat per ounce) • All natural cheeses, low-fat or Sherbet or sorbet, nonfat ice cream or "light" cream cheese & sour cream frozen yogurt	• Whole or 2% milk, half & half, imitation milk products or creamers & whipped Low-fat cheeses, farmer cheese, pot cheeses toppings. • Whole-milk yogurt & cottage • Ice cream
Eggs	
• Egg whites (2 whites = 1 whole egg in recipes) • cholesterol-free egg substitutes	• Egg yolks

HOW TO READ NUTRITION FACTS LABELS

When mixing up your meals, the Nutrition Facts labels can help you make smart choices about the variety of foods in your eating program.

Food label guide

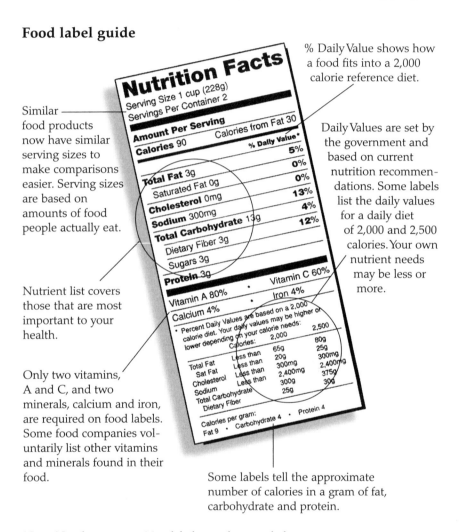

Similar food products now have similar serving sizes to make comparisons easier. Serving sizes are based on amounts of food people actually eat.

Nutrient list covers those that are most important to your health.

Only two vitamins, A and C, and two minerals, calcium and iron, are required on food labels. Some food companies voluntarily list other vitamins and minerals found in their food.

% Daily Value shows how a food fits into a 2,000 calorie reference diet.

Daily Values are set by the government and based on current nutrition recommendations. Some labels list the daily values for a daily diet of 2,000 and 2,500 calories. Your own nutrient needs may be less or more.

Some labels tell the approximate number of calories in a gram of fat, carbohydrate and protein.

Note: Numbers on nutrition labels may be rounded.

The U.S. Food and Drug Administration's Center for Food Safety and Applied Nutrition provides an even more detailed breakdown of these labels (*www.cfsan.fda.gov*).

Serving Size: Lists standard amount an individual would consume in a single serving in common units (cups, numbers of pieces, etc.).

Percent Daily Value: Indicates how the product figures into a 2,000-calorie diet; yet, it can sill be used as a frame of reference if you consume more or less than 2,000 calories.

Central Nutrition Panel: Lists the nutrients that are most important to good health. Helps you calculate your daily limits for fat, fiber, sodium and your daily intake of other nutrients like carbohydrates and proteins.

Vitamins & Minerals: Lists the Percent Daily Value, which is the same as the U.S. Recommended Daily Allowance for vitamins and minerals (same levels). Only Vitamin A, Vitamin C, Calcium and Iron are required on labels, although manufacturers have the option to include other vitamins and minerals as well.

Footnote: Lists reference values for good nutrition basics. Can be adjusted to fit an individual's caloric needs.

RULE 2 • Get Carb Smart!

THE GLYCEMIC INDEX

The Glycemic Index measures how fast foods raise your blood sugar. GI's are based on glucose (GI 100), the fastest carb. Fast carbs (high numbers) help to raise low blood sugars for short periods of intense exercise. Slow carbs (low numbers) prevent overnight drops in blood sugar and during long periods of exercise. The impact of foods on blood sugar depends on factors like ripeness, cooking time, fiber and fat content, time of day, blood insulin levels and recent activity.

Glucose scores 100. Foods less than 55 are low. Foods above 70 are high. Foods that fall between 55 and 70 are medium. Generally, high-glycemic carbs promote a rapid glucose spike, followed by an insulin spike, which sends the sugar into the cells. The result is a corresponding drop in blood sugar, a lack of energy and increased hunger sooner rather than later. Low-glycemic carbs provide a slower glucose rise and a more sustained energy level.

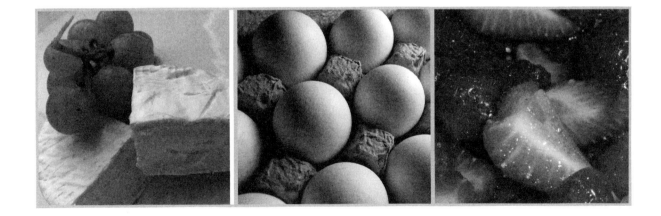

Glycemic Index Chart

Beans

baby lima 32
baked 43
black 30
brown 38
butter 31
chickpeas 33
kidney 27
lentil 30
navy 38
pinto 42
red lentils 27
split peas 32
soy 18

Breads

bagel 72
croissant 67
Kaiser roll 73
pita 57
pumpernickel 49
rye 64
rye, dark 76
rye, whole 50
white 72
whole wheat 72
waffles 76

Cereals

Bran 44
Cheerios 74
Corn Bran 75
Corn Chex 83
Cornflakes 83
Cream of Wheat 66
Crispix 87
Frosted Flakes 55
Grapenuts 67
NutriGrain 66
Oatmeal 49
Puffed Wheat 74
Rice Krispies 82
Shredded Wheat 69
Special K 54
Total 76

Cookies

Graham crackers 74
oatmeal 55
shortbread 64
Vanilla Wafers 77

Crackers

rice cakes 82
rye 63
saltine 72
wheat thins 67
water crackers 78

Desserts

angel food cake 67a
banana bread 47
blueberry muffin 59
bran muffin 60
Danish 59
fruit bread 47
pound cake 54
sponge cake 46
ice cream 50
pudding 43

Fruit

apple 38
apricot, canned 64
apricot, dried 30
banana 62
cantaloupe 65
cherries 22
dates, dried 103
fruit cocktail 55
grapefruit 25
grapes 43
kiwi 52
chickpeas 36
orange 43
papaya 58
peach 42
pear 36
pineapple 66
plum 24
raisins 64
strawberries 32
watermelon 72

Grains

barley 22
brown rice 59
buckwheat 54
mac & cheese 64
cornmeal 68
couscous 65
hominy 40
rice, instant 91
rice, parboiled 47
rye 34
sweet corn 55
wheat, whole 41
white rice 88

Juices

gave nectar 11
apple 41
grapefruit 48
orange 55
pineapple 46

Milk Products

chocolate milk 34
milk 34
soy milk 31
yogurt 38

Pasta

brown pasta 92
linguine 50
macaroni 46
spaghetti 40
vermicelli 35

Sweets

honey 58
jelly beans 80
hard candy 70
chocolate bar 41

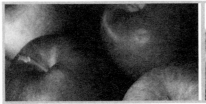
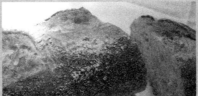
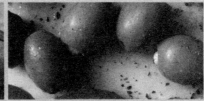

RULE 3 • Avoid Bad Fat!

Although *all* fats are concentrated sources of calories and can contribute to weight gain (and thus, high blood cholesterol levels), *saturated fat* is the most harmful type. Saturated fat is the main cause of high blood cholesterol levels. When you eat too much saturated fat, your body reacts by making more cholesterol than it needs, and the surplus ends up in your blood. Both monounsaturated and polyunsaturated fats help lower blood cholesterol levels by helping your body get rid of newly formed cholesterol.

THE DIFFERENCE BETWEEN LDL AND HDL CHOLESTEROL*

Why is LDL cholesterol considered "bad"?

When too much LDL cholesterol circulates in the blood, it can slowly build up in the inner walls of the arteries that feed the heart and brain. Together with other substances, it can form plaque, a thick, hard deposit that can clog those arteries. This condition is known as atherosclerosis. If a clot forms and blocks a narrowed artery, it can cause a heart attack or stroke. The levels of HDL and LDL blood cholesterol are measured to evaluate the risk of a heart attack. LDL cholesterol of less than 100 mg/dL is the optimal level. Less than 130 mg/dL is near optimal for most people. A high LDL level (more than 160 mg/dL or 130 mg/dL or above if you have two or more risk factors for cardiovascular disease) reflects an increased risk of heart disease. That's why LDL cholesterol is often called "bad" cholesterol.

Why is HDL cholesterol considered "good"?

About one-third to one-fourth of blood cholesterol is carried by high-density lipoprotein (HDL). HDL cholesterol is known as the "good" cholesterol because a high level of it seems to protect against heart attack. (Low HDL cholesterol levels [less than 40 mg/dL] increase the risk for heart disease.) Medical experts think that HDL tends to carry cholesterol away from the arteries and back to the liver, where it's passed from the body. Some experts believe HDL removes excess cholesterol from plaque in arteries, thus slowing the buildup.

---

* *(Consult your physician for a full explanation of cholesterol and to measure your levels.)*

(According to the American Heart Association www.americanheart.org)

RULE 3 • Burn Your Food!

Here are *5 REAL Keys to Weight Management* to help you identify calorie-burning practices versus calorie-storing practices.

1. INCREASE VERSUS DECREASE
   Increase daily physical activity, while you decrease daily caloric intake (as needed).

2. ACCESS VERSUS RECESS
   Monitor access to food and duration of recess (inactive rest); get just enough of both to maintain health.

3. QUALITY VERSUS QUANTITY
   Consume balanced, quality meals, and avoid diets involving extreme quantities, i.e., starving *or* gorging.

4. MODERATION VERSUS ELIMINATION
   Use moderation and portion control as opposed to skipping meals or eliminating foods.

5. CHANGE VERSUS TREND
   Adopt lifestyle and eating changes that last a lifetime versus short-lived diet and fitness trends.

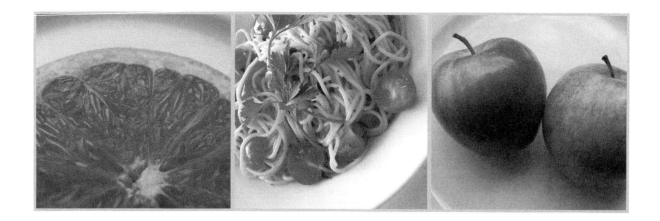

THE REAL SMART SHOPPER'S GROCERY CHECKLIST

Now that you have reviewed how to put together your *REAL DEAL Meal Plan*, use the following checklist of tips to navigate through the grocery store and make healthy choices in selecting the foods you need to make your eating program a success.

Where to shop • Bakery Department

☐ **What to buy** • Pick whole-wheat or whole-grain breads, bagels and English muffins. Avoid sweetened pastries, doughnuts, muffins, cakes and croissants.

Where to shop • Dairy Department

☐ **What to buy** • Pick low-fat or fat-free milk, cheese, cottage cheese, yogurt and margarine.

Where to shop • Deli/Meat Department

☐ **What to buy** • Pick fresh fish, lean beef, skinless chicken and turkey, pre-roasted chicken, tenderloin pork and low-fat, low-sodium luncheon meat. Avoid fatty sausage, bacon and hot dogs.

Where to shop • Frozen Foods Department

☐ **What to buy** • Pick low-fat, low-sodium frozen breakfasts, dinners, microwaveable meals, entrees, soups, side dishes, snacks, mixed berries, mixed veggies, sorbet, juice bars and yogurt.

Where to shop • Packaged Foods Department

☐ **What to buy** • Pick low-fat peanut butter and condiments. Pick low-fat, low-sodium canned soups, fruits (in their own juices), vegetables, meats and tuna (in water). Pick whole-grain, low-sugar, low-fat, low-sodium cereals, crackers, pastas and rice.

Where to shop • Produce Department

☐ **What to buy** • Pick produce in a wide variety of colors and types and convenient pre-cut/pre-bagged fruits and veggies.

REAL DEAL EATING LOG

Track your REAL DEAL meals and daily caloric intake.

These are basic principles to keep in mind as you plan your eating program:

Basic Real Deal Nutrition Principles

Rev up your water intake.
Enjoy protein-rich, carb-smart foods.
Add a multivitamin to supplement your diet.
Limit your intake of fat, sugar & sodium.

Date: _____/_____/_____

Day: M T W Th F Sat Sun *(circle one)*   Time:_____

Breakfast:

Meal Time:_____

Calories (optional):_____

Meal Contents:_____

Snack:

Meal Time:_____

Calories (optional):_____

Meal Contents:_____

Lunch:

Meal Time:_____

Calories (optional):_____

Meal Contents:_____

Snack:

Meal Time:_____

Calories (optional):_____

Meal Contents:_____

Dinner:

Meal Time:_____

Calories (optional):_____

Meal Contents:_____

Notes:

Daily Multivitamin?_____ *(check reminder)*

Total Calories Consumed (optional):_____

Miscellaneous Notes:_____
_____
_____

(Make photocopies of this page, collect them for your records and refer to them as a motivational tool.)

ABOUT THE AUTHORS

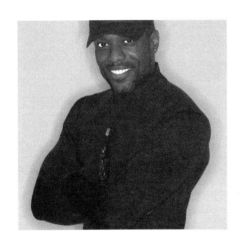

COACH ANDREW OYE

Andrew Oye is a Certified Fitness Trainer, specializing in Strength & Conditioning, Toning and Sport-Specific Training. Andrew has developed personalized training programs to meet the various fitness goals of a range of clients at large sports clubs and small private studios. Andrew has also trained amateur natural bodybuilders for competition. Andrew earned a Bachelor's of Science in Human & Organizational Development from Vanderbilt University. Andrew served as an Athletic Trainer Intern at the Vanderbilt University Sports Medicine Clinic, assisting the staff with the physical rehabilitation/treatment programs of athletes. Andrew assisted with the launch of a weight-loss and fitness program at Emory-Adventist Hospital. Andrew earned a Master's of Art in Communications from Stanford University. The former Creative & Editorial Director of BUILT Magazine, Andrew is a fitness and bodybuilding industry journalist and his writing has appeared on bodybuilding.com, myfittribe.com, prosource.net and in Planet Muscle Magazine. He is the creator of the "The Oye Body Survey," a popular profile survey for fitness enthusiasts. A novelist, screenwriter and creative strategist, Andrew's communications experience includes executing PR and marketing campaigns for sports/entertainment clients and providing editorial consultation to sports nutrition firms.

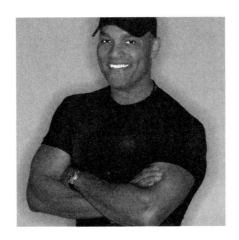

COACH ROBERT DOTHARD

Robert Dothard is a Certified Personal Trainer and Group Exercise Instructor, a motivational speaker and a Black Belt level trainer in Tae Kwon Do. Currently hosting the "Wakeup Workout" segments on NBC's 11-Alive newscast, Robert has also shared his fitness expertise and wellness philosophy via segments on CNN and affiliates of ABC, CBS and FOX Networks. Robert earned a Bachelor's of Arts in Business Administration at LaGrange College. Robert has recruited for such companies as Sports Life®, opened the first Gold's Gym® in Georgia, was a representative for Crunch®, Australian Body Works (now L.A. Fitness®) and now owns two Fitness Together training studios. A fitness pioneer, Robert was the first male Step Aerobics Instructor in history. In 1996, Robert served as the Step Aerobics Instructor and Personal Trainer for Olympic athletes during the Centennial Olympic Summer Games in Atlanta. Robert has appeared in the RAMP Video Series with the creator of Step Aerobics, Gin Miller, and has endorsed several exercise and fitness products (BodyTrends.com, Heavy Hands™, and Polar BodyAge™). More information on Robert is available at www.robertdothard.com.

NOTES

NOTES

NOTES

NOTES